national
STATISTICS

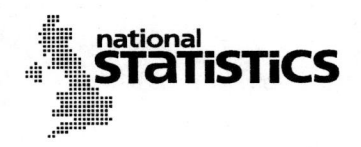

Series MB1 no. 32

Cancer statistics registrations

Registrations of cancer diagnosed in 2001, England

London: Office for National Statistics

© Crown copyright 2004
Published with the permission of the Controller of Her Majesty's Stationery Office (HMSO)

ISBN 1 85774 587 6
ISSN 0143–4829

This publication, excluding logos, may be reproduced free of charge, in any format or medium for research or private study subject to it being reproduced accurately and not used in a misleading context. The material must be acknowledged as crown copyright and the title of the publication specified. This publication can also be accessed at the National Statistics website: www.statistics.gov.uk

For any other use of this material please apply for a free Click-Use Licence on the HMSO website:
www.hmso.gov.uk/click-use-home.htm
Or write to HMSO at The Licensing Division, St Clement's House, 2-16 Colegate, Norwich NR3 1BQ. Fax 01603 723000 or e-mail: hmsolicencing@cabinetoffice.x.gsi.gov.uk

Contact points
For enquiries about this publication, contact the Editors:
Helen Booth
Mark Gautrey
Margaret Sheldrake
Nicola Cooper
Dr Mike Quinn
Tel: 01329 813620
E-mail: mark.gautrey@ons.gsi.gov.uk

For general enquiries, contact the National Statistics Customer Contact Centre on: 0845 601 3034
(minicom: 01633 812399)
E-mail: info@statistics.gsi.gov.uk
Fax: 01633 652747
Post: Room 1015, Government Buildings,
Cardiff Road, Newport NP10 8XG

You can also find National Statistics on the Internet at:
www.statistics.gov.uk

About the Office for National Statistics
The Office for National Statistics (ONS) is the government agency responsible for compiling, analysing and disseminating many of the United Kingdom's economic, social and demographic statistics, including the retail prices index, trade figures and labour market data, as well as the periodic census of the population and health statistics. It is also the agency that administers the statutory registration of births, marriages and deaths in England and Wales. The Director of ONS is also the National Statistician and the Registrar General for England and Wales.

A National Statistics publication
National Statistics are produced to high professional standards set out in the National Statistics Code of Practice. They undergo regular quality assurance reviews to ensure that they meet customer needs. They are produced free from any political influence.

Contents

	Page
List of tables	iv
Introduction	1
Background	1
Cancer registration system	1
Acknowledgements	2
Outline of contents	2
Cancer registration in England and Wales	4
The United Kingdom Association of Cancer Registries	11
Cancer registrations, 2001	13
Cumulative risk of cancer	16
Cancer incidence in the UK, 1999-2001	16
Tables (see page iv)	18
Appendix 1 Guidance notes and definitions	64
1 Data	64
Cancer registrations	64
Quality of cancer registration data	64
Mortality data	68
Quality of mortality data	69
Advantages and disadvantages of incidence and mortality data	69
Populations	70
Government Offices for the Regions (GORs)	70
2 Methods	70
Age standardised rates	70
Cumulative lifetime risk	71
Survival	71
Symbols and conventions used	71
Further information	71
Appendix 2 Maps and contact addresses	74

List of tables

			Page
Table 1	Registrations of newly diagnosed cases of cancer (3rd digit): site, sex and age, 2001	England	18
Table 2	Estimated resident population: sex and age, as at 30 June 2001	England and government office for the region	28
Table 3	Rates per 100,000 population of newly diagnosed cases of cancer (3rd digit): site, sex and age, 2001	England	30
Table 4	Registrations of newly diagnosed cases of cancer (3rd digit): site, sex and government office for the region of residence, 2001	England and government office for the region	40
Table 5	Rates per 100,000 population of newly diagnosed cases of cancer (3rd digit): site, sex and government office for the region of residence, 2001	England and government office for the region	45
Table 6	Standardised registration ratios: site, sex and government office for the region of residence, 2001 (England = 100)	Government office for the region	50
Table 7	Registrations of newly diagnosed cases of cancer (4th digit): site, sex and age, 2001	England	*
Table 8	Rates per 100,000 population of newly diagnosed cases of cancer (4th digit): site, sex and age, 2001	England	*
Table 9	Cancer mortality to incidence ratios: site, sex and government office for the region of residence, 2001	England and government office for the region	55
Table 10	Directly age standardised registration rates per 100,000 population: site and sex, 1992 to 2001	England	59

* These large tables are available on the National Statistics website: www.statistics.gov.uk

Introduction

Cancer statistics - registrations 2001 presents data for England on those patients who were diagnosed with cancer during 2001 and whose registrations were received at the Office for National Statistics (ONS) by the end of May 2004.

At the beginning of April 1996, the Office of Population Censuses and Surveys (OPCS) merged with the Central Statistical Office (CSO) to form the ONS. ONS is responsible for the full range of functions previously carried out by CSO and OPCS, including labour market statistics and registration of births, marriages and deaths. Whilst ONS is responsible for assembling and disseminating UK statistics, no functions held by Scottish or Northern Irish Departments have been transferred to ONS. Previous volumes in this series up to no.27 (1994)[1] have presented data for England and Wales. This volume, as did nos. 28 to 31[2-5] covers only England, because all matters relating to health in Wales have been devolved to the National Assembly of Wales (NAW). Cancer registration in Wales is carried out by the Welsh Cancer Intelligence and Surveillance Unit (WCISU) under a service level agreement with the NAW, the terms of which are closely similar to those in the national standards for cancer registration in England. The WCISU is a member of the UK Association of Cancer Registries (UKACR - see below) and voluntarily adheres to all the UKACR's agreed standards and guidelines.

Comparable statistics for England and Wales for 1971 to 1994 have been published in the *Cancer statistics - registrations* (Series MB1) reports. A CD-ROM[6] is also available from ONS containing anonymised records of new cases diagnosed from 1971 to 1992 and deaths from cancer from 1971 to 1997, in England and Wales (see page 69); an update to this, covering the 1990s will be available in the autumn of 2004. For years prior to 1971, statistics have been published in the *Registrar General's Statistical Review of England and Wales, Supplements on Cancer.*

In February 2000 ONS published the book *Cancer Trends in England and Wales 1950-1999*[7]. This brought together for the first time the long term trends in cancer incidence, mortality, prevalence and survival for all the major cancers (which together make up almost 90% of the total cases in both males and females) accompanied by brief notes on aetiology and risk factors. New analyses, based on data for the whole population, highlight the wide variations in cancer incidence and mortality with socio-economic deprivation. The book paints the broad picture of the cancer burden and illustrates the baselines against which progress in cancer control will be measured.

Background

Marked changes in the incidence of, and mortality from, cancer have occurred since the beginning of this century. Currently, about one person in three in England develops a cancer sometime in their life, and cancer now causes about one in four deaths. Around 320,000 new cases of cancer are registered every year, and there are about 135,000 deaths from cancer.

It has been estimated that the treatment of cancer accounts for 6 per cent of all NHS hospital expenditure, amounting to over £1 billion a year.[8] Support for research into cancer in the late 1990s was over £260 million each year; total government expenditure amounted to around £25 million, while spending by charities totalled around £125 million and that by the pharmaceutical industry over £110 million.[9]

Key people involved in cancer prevention and control include scientists investigating the mechanisms which cause cells to become malignant; those carrying out clinical trials to evaluate new treatments; clinicians treating individual patients; public health physicians implementing screening programmes and educating the public; and epidemiologists attempting to characterise high- and low-risk populations, identify causal factors and provide clues to carcinogenic mechanisms.

Evaluation of this work in any coherent way requires a population-based cancer surveillance system which can monitor variations in incidence and survival over time, between places and between different groups in the population. The NHS Cancer Plan[10] published in 2000 recognised the key role of the cancer registries.

Cancer registration system

Questions seeking information for the purposes of cancer registration in England and Wales were first asked in the 1920s; a national scheme has been in existence since 1945 - initially centred on the Radium Commission, but from 1947 onwards at the General Register Office, and at its successors, OPCS and, since April 1996, ONS. Complete geographic national coverage was achieved in 1962. Cancer registration is now conducted by nine independent regional registries in England which collect, on a voluntary basis, data on cancers incident in residents of their areas, and submit a standard data set on these registrations to ONS. In England, each of the regional health authority (RHA) areas which existed in

1994 was covered by its own cancer registry - except that all four Thames RHAs were covered by one registry. As a result of subsequent changes to administrative boundaries in the NHS, together with mergers of some regional cancer registries, by 2001 when the health regions were abolished, the only registry whose area was fully coterminous with a health region boundary was the West Midlands Cancer Intelligence Unit based in Birmingham. A map showing the areas covered by the nine cancer registries is given in Appendix 2. As noted above, the NAW is now responsible for cancer registration in Wales. A fuller description of the scheme is given below.

Under similar arrangements there is a system of cancer registration in Scotland, co-ordinated by the Information and Statistics Division (ISD) of the NHS in Scotland Common Services Agency in Edinburgh. The Scottish Cancer Registry is a full member of the UKACR. ONS and the regional registries in England maintain close contacts with the Welsh Cancer Intelligence and Surveillance Unit, the Scottish Cancer Registry and the Northern Ireland Cancer Registry, and co-operate in several areas, including answering Parliamentary Questions relating to Great Britain or the UK; supplying information for projects such as the preparation of a cancer atlas, and for the examination of clusters of disease by the Small Area Health Statistics Unit at the Imperial College School of Medicine at St Mary's; and assisting the charity Cancer Research UK with information for its UK-based 'CancerStats'. The book *Cancer Trends in England and Wales 1950-1999*[7] also contains some key cancer statistics on the major sites for the UK, and each of the 20 site specific chapters contains a summary table with information for all the regions of England and for Wales, Scotland and Northern Ireland.

Acknowledgements

It is with gratitude that ONS acknowledges the work of the regional cancer registries over the years that the national scheme has been in operation, and their close co-operation with the national registry. The full addresses, telephone and fax numbers of the registries in England, and the registries in Wales, Scotland and Northern Ireland, are given in Appendix 2. The current directors of the registries in England are:

Northern & Yorkshire	Professor R Haward (Medical Director)
	Professor D Forman (Director of Information and Research)
Trent	Post vacant
East Anglian	Dr J Rashbass (General Director)
	Dr C H Brown (Medical Director)
Thames	Professor H Møller
South & West	Dr J Verne (Acting Director)
Oxford	Dr M Roche
West Midlands	Dr G Lawrence
Merseyside & Cheshire	Dr E M I Williams
North Western	Dr A Moran

Outline of contents

Notes on the change of coverage to England are given above. The cancer site codes and descriptions reflect the adoption by the NHS in 1995 of the 10th Revision of the International Statistical Classification of Diseases and Related Health Problems (ICD10).[11] **Table 1** contains the numbers of newly diagnosed cases of cancer by site to the 3rd digit of the ICD10 code, sex and five year age group. **Table 2** presents population estimates by sex and five year age group for 2001, based on the 1991 census. **Table 3** gives the rates of cancer incidence per 100,000 population by sex and five year age group corresponding to the numbers of cases in Table 1. **Table 4** gives the numbers of cancer registrations and **Table 5** the rates per 100,000 population by sex and government office for the region (GOR). **Table 6** gives the standardised registration ratios by GOR by site and sex (England as base). **Table 7 and 8** present the numbers and rates per 100,000 population respectively, of newly diagnosed cases of cancer, by site to the 4th digit of the ICD10 code, sex and age group. These very large tables are not included in this volume, but are available on the National Statistics website: **www.statistics.gov.uk**. **Table 9** contains cancer mortality to incidence ratios by site, sex and GOR. **Table 10** gives the directly age standardised rates per 100,000 population, using the European standard population, of new cancer cases for England for the 10 year period 1992-2001 by site and sex. Data have been aggregated by cancer sub-site where necessary to give consistent time series across the change in coding in 1995 from ICD9[12] to ICD10.

The commentary which follows begins with a brief history of the scheme, covering the four reviews of the system published in 1970, 1980, 1990 and 2001; the role of ONS; and the setting up of the National Steering Committee on Cancer Registration (subsequently the Advisory Committee). Also described is the establishment of the United Kingdom Association of Cancer Registries. The next sections give the overall results for all cancer sites in 2001, estimates of the cumulative (lifetime) risk of cancer, and figures of the incidence of the 20 or so most common cancers in the UK. Following these are the detailed tables described above. Finally, appendices contain guidance notes and definitions and a discussion of some factors relevant to the interpretation of cancer registration data, and information on the cancer registries.

References

1. ONS. *Cancer statistics - registrations, England and Wales, 1994*. Series MB1 no.27. London: The Stationery Office, 2000.
2. ONS. *Cancer statistics - registrations, England, 1995-1997*. Series MB1 no.28. London: The Stationery Office, 2001.
3. ONS. *Cancer statistics - registrations, England, 1998*. Series MB1 no. 29. London: Office for National Statistics, 2001.

4. ONS. *Cancer statistics - registrations, England, 1999.* Series MB1 no. 30. London: Office for National Statistics, 2002.
5. ONS. *Cancer statistics - registrations, England, 2000.* Series MB1 no. 31. London: Office for National Statistics, 2003.
6. Quinn MJ, Babb PJ, Jones J, Baker A, Ault C. *Cancer 1971-1997.* Registrations of cancer cases and deaths in England and Wales by sex, age, year, health region and type of cancer (CD-ROM). London: Office for National Statistics, 1999.
7. Quinn MJ, Babb P, Brock A, Kirby L, Jones J. *Cancer Trends in England and Wales 1950-1999.* Studies in Medical and Population Subjects No.66. London: The Stationery Office, 2001.
8. *A policy framework for commissioning cancer services.* A report by the Expert Advisory Group on cancer to the Chief Medical Officers of England and Wales. London: Department of Health and Welsh Office, 1995.
9. NHS Executive. *Expenditure on cancer research 1995/96.* Leeds: NHS Executive, 1996.
10. Department of Health. *The NHS Cancer Plan.* London: Department of Health, 2000.
11. World Health Organisation. *International Statistical Classification of Diseases and Related Health Problems - Tenth Revision.* Geneva: WHO, 1992.
12. World Health Organisation. *International Classification of Diseases - Ninth Revision.* Geneva: WHO, 1977.

Cancer registration in England and Wales

This chapter presents a brief history of the cancer registration system in England and Wales and an outline of the role of the Office for National Statistics (ONS).

Background and early history

Cancer registration is the process of maintaining a systematic collection of data on the occurrence and characteristics of malignant neoplasms and certain non-malignant tumours. The procedure is widely established throughout the world and generally follows guidelines established by bodies such as the International Union Against Cancer (UICC), the International Agency for Research on Cancer (IARC), the International Association of Cancer Registries (IACR), and the World Health Organisation (WHO)[1,2].

The great and increasing suffering due to cancer was of concern to the Ministry of Health in the early 1920s and with the introduction of radium treatment, a system was initiated in parts of England and Wales to follow the outcome of treated patients. Both the Radium Commission of 1929 and the Cancer Act of 1939 (never implemented because of the war) incorporated the principle that statistical information about cancer patients was essential for planning and operating cancer care services. In 1945, the Radium Commission was designated as the Statistical Bureau to which the data should be sent for final analysis. This work was taken over by the General Register Office in 1947; and the Cancer Act was repealed in 1948 when the National Health Service Act came into force. From that time the General Register Office, its successors OPCS and, more recently, ONS, have collected and processed data forwarded under voluntary arrangements. Since January 1993, it has been mandatory for the NHS, including trusts, to provide the core items listed in the cancer registration minimum data set to the regional cancer registries; and for the registries to send these data to ONS (see page 6).

The 1960s

In February 1963 a conference was held at the Ministry of Health for the purposes of paving the way for 100 per cent registration of cancer patients and for seeking means of improving the cancer registration scheme. A Working Party agreed on the regional and national objectives of the cancer registration scheme. At the **regional** level, the objectives were to improve the service to the cancer patient through good record keeping and efficient follow-up; and to provide information for local research into the value of treatment and for epidemiological studies, for the planning and assessment of the cancer service, and for the production of national statistics. At the **national** level, the objectives were to produce national statistical analyses likely to assist in the management of the disease and the understanding of it; to cooperate with other Government Departments and outside bodies in any survey aimed at furthering knowledge of the disease; and to participate, by supplying statistical data as required, in the work of international cancer organisations established to carry out research into the cause and course of cancer.

The Working Party spent a considerable amount of time determining what information should be obtained for analysis at the national level, but it was agreed that the information requested should be kept to a minimum - with the intention of obtaining a more complete record and a greater degree of accuracy. The Working Party's report also discussed and agreed recommendations on desirable national and regional tabulations; the elimination of duplicate activity (in data processing); duplicate registrations; dissemination of information; and the unique difficulties of the (then) Metropolitan Regional Hospital Board areas which are now covered by the Thames registry and the office of South and West Cancer Intelligence Service in Winchester (formerly the Wessex registry).

Advisory Committee Report 1970

Following discussions in 1969 between the Department of Health and Social Security (DHSS) and the Registrar General, an Advisory Committee on Cancer Registration was set up. It was requested simply 'to consider and advise on matters of policy and method relating to the national cancer registration scheme', and its members included several eminent epidemiologists in addition to representatives from the DHSS, the registries and (the then) OPCS.

The Committee reviewed the existing scheme, in which each case of cancer was registered first of all on a registration form and the data subsequently transferred onto an abstract card. These were to be updated and resubmitted to OPCS after five, ten and fifteen years. Each registry received, through the machinery of the general system of vital registration and statistics, details of any death in its area where cancer was mentioned on the death certificate (this is known as the 'green card' system after the colour of the paper onto which the death certificate information was copied). Much difficulty had been caused at OPCS by the late submission of abstract cards, and - even worse - of follow-up cards. The quality of data varied considerably among the regions and even the best fell 'rather short' of 100 per cent accuracy in all particulars. The Committee felt that some of the data collected (for example on treatment) were of doubtful value and placed an unnecessary workload on the registries.

There was, however, unanimous agreement that some form of national cancer registration scheme was necessary in order not only to establish national incidence rates and monitor them for purposes of logistic planning and general epidemiological research, but also to permit prospective studies of cancer in selected groups of the population. In addition, information at the international level for comparison with experience in other countries made a valuable contribution to the understanding of the disease.

Revised scheme

A revised scheme was proposed[3], covering the definition of cases to be registered; the documentation (a revised and shortened abstract card); a nominal index for use by research workers; national tabulations (to be produced by OPCS); and death notifications (green cards). Probably the most important change suggested was that the system of five, ten and fifteen year follow-up abstract cards should be stopped. Instead, cancer registrations would be 'flagged' in the records maintained by the National Health Service Central Register (NHSCR) - another part of OPCS - in Southport, in the same way that deaths were. As non-cancer deaths of persons flagged as cancer-registered could be notified routinely to the registries, this, together with the green cards, would relieve them of the expensive and laborious task of tracing patients clerically (for example by using hospital records or writing to GPs). This revised scheme was introduced in 1971, backdated to cover all registrations whose anniversary date fell on or after 1 January 1971. The essential features of the system (illustrated in Figure A) have now remained unchanged for over 30 years.

Advisory Committee Report 1980

The revised scheme was reviewed some ten years later when the Advisory Committee was reconvened. Its report[4] presented a large amount of national statistics on cancer incidence, survival, prevalence and mortality. It also highlighted the growing demands for information for clinical research; planning, organising and evaluating services for the prevention and treatment of cancer; epidemiological research; and education of the public.

Many of the Committee's comments on areas where problems were being experienced are still relevant today. The Committee re-emphasised the great value of recording the NHS number, and stressed that personal identification data were essential - for the elimination of duplicate notifications, to enable follow-up and calculation of survival rates, and to enable registrations data to be linked (with suitable safeguards) to other data about the same person. They found a substantial degree of variation among the regions in the excess of registrations over deaths; although difficult to interpret, this suggested an equivalent variation in the degree of ascertainment. The report discussed the three main methods of collection: peripatetic staff, hospital staff and the Hospital Activity Analysis (HAA) system. HAA data were often considered to be insufficiently reliable, but the Committee noted that the three registries which used HAA as their primary source were not those which had low numbers of registrations compared with deaths. The use of information from pathology departments, to increase not only the accuracy but also the completeness of ascertainment, was encouraged. As well as being complete, the data needed to be up to date

Figure A The cancer registration system of England and Wales

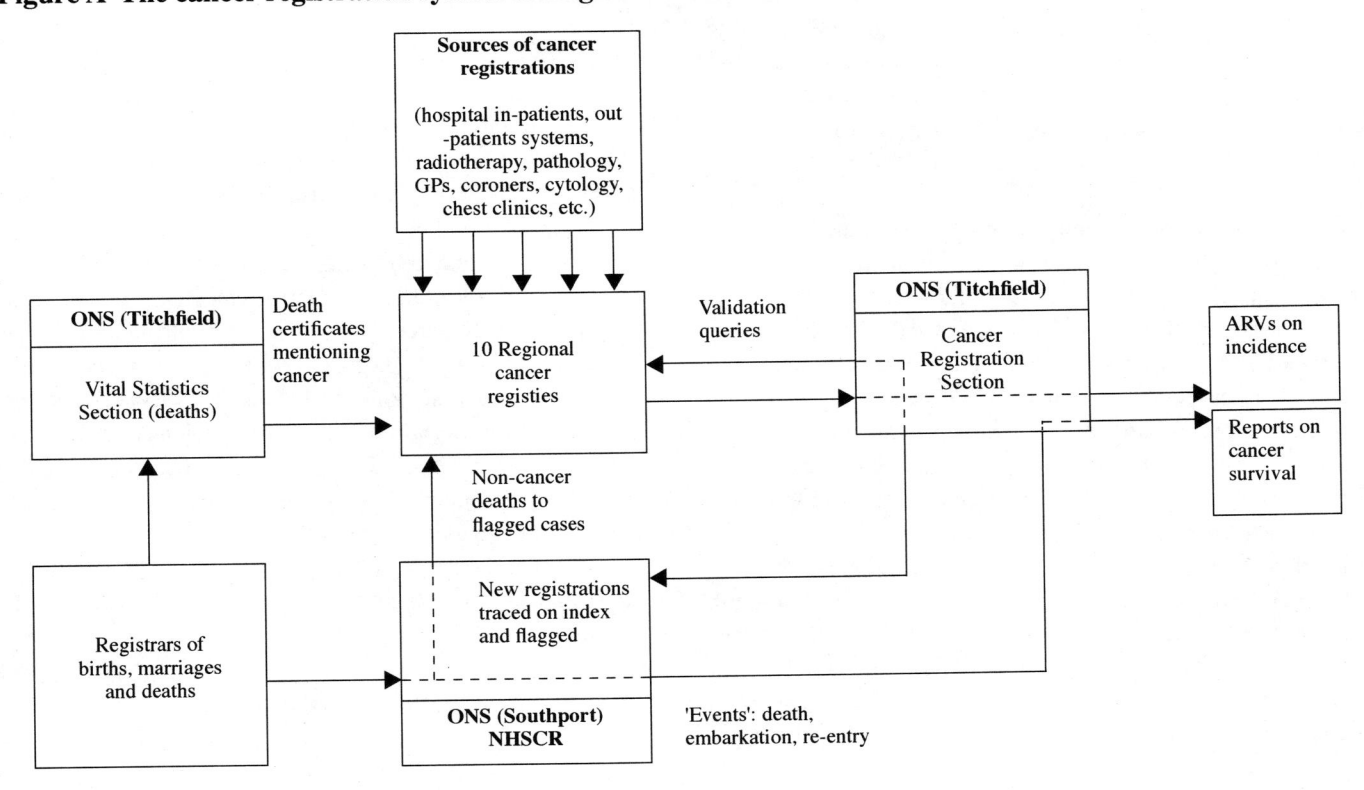

and here the Committee found grave shortcomings since the inception of the revised scheme.

While the average cost of registering one patient with cancer was only a very small fraction of the total cost of the management of the patient's illness, it was noted that (in England) the regional registries were funded by the regional health authorities, with no direct financial input from the DHSS or OPCS. It was possible that registration might not be given the necessary resources at regional level where priorities were decided autonomously.

The Committee concluded that cancer registration covering the whole of England and Wales should continue and be improved in several areas for the following reasons: preventative action was usually based on information from epidemiological studies (using the national register linked to the NHSCR); changes in incidence needed to be monitored because of public, political and medical concern, and improvements in treatment were making mortality data increasingly unreliable as an index of trends; changes in survival needed to be monitored; and reliable and up-to-date data on incidence were essential for the planning and operating of services for cancer detection and treatment.

Medical Advisory Committee review 1990

In 1989 a Working Group of the Registrar General's Medical Advisory Committee (MAC) was set up to review the operation of the cancer registration system, particularly the regional and national data collection methods, the quality and timeliness of the statistics produced, the uses made of the regional and national registers, and the growing tendency to treat cancers in out-patient departments or privately. It was also asked to consider the implications of changes in demand for information and developments in information technology, and the priorities and level of resources required to maintain adequate registers. The potential implications of the recommendations of the White Paper *Working for Patients*[5] were also considered.

The Working Group[6] noted that in addition to the traditional uses of cancer registration (monitoring of time trends and geographical variation in incidence), the system had become vital in several other areas. These included the management of the substantial resources required for the preventative, curative and laboratory services for cancer; the planning and evaluation of services, particularly the screening programmes for breast and cervical cancer; the planning and evaluation of clinical management and treatment based on accurate and unbiased survival data and clinical trials; research into causes of cancer, involving case-control studies and the flagging of cohorts at the NHSCR; and information for health education and health promotion for both professionals and the public. Future uses of cancer registration (especially if linked with other databases) were identified, including evaluating programmes of care, quality assurance, and relating costs to clinical outcome.

The seventeen recommendations made by the Working Group for improvements to the system fell into several categories, relating to the organisation of the system; the collection, processing, quality, timeliness and completeness of the data; and the safeguarding of the necessary data release in view of the impending NHS changes and the growing use of the private sector.

One of the six recommendations in the 'organisational' area was that a Steering Committee should be established to oversee national cancer registration, with representation from the registries, OPCS, regional and district health authorities, the UK Co-ordinating Committee of Cancer Research, the Health and Safety Executive and the private health sector. This Steering Committee, which was chaired by Dr J Metters, the Deputy Chief Medical Officer at the Department of Health, held its first meeting in June 1991 and met subsequently at approximately six monthly intervals. This committee was re-formed as the Advisory Committee on Cancer Registration; it was chaired by Dr S Atkinson of the NHS Executive.

Three recommendations involved both the registries and OPCS: an expanded national core data set; co-operation with the private health sector; and the establishment of guidelines for the handling and release of data. These have been discussed at several consultative meetings with the registries. Work on three other recommendations, relating to the provision of timely estimates of incidence at the national and regional level, quality control checks and the provision of up-to-date anonymous and summary data, was carried forward at ONS which in 1995 completed the redevelopment of its longstanding computer system to a new database environment (see below).

The role of ONS in cancer registration

The Office for National Statistics was formed by the merger of OPCS and the Central Statistical Office (CSO) in 1996. The Director of ONS, Mr Len Cook, is also the Registrar General for England and Wales. The National Cancer Intelligence Centre (NCIC) at ONS includes part of the Health and Care Division in London which co-ordinates all the work on cancer registration and carries out a wide range of secondary analysis and research; part of the Social Data Collection and Administrative Sources Division in Titchfield which conducts the primary data processing of registry data; and a section at the NHSCR in Southport which flags the cancer registrations on the central register. Much of the secondary analysis and research, which is carried out by a statistician and three researchers, supported by a medical epidemiologist and a Professor of Epidemiology and Vital Statistics at the London School of Hygiene and Tropical Medicine (LSHTM), is done in collaboration with academic and external researchers, for example at the LSHTM, the Cancer Screening Evaluation Unit at the Institute for Cancer Research, and the Small Area Health Statistics Unit at Imperial College.

Most registries collect a large amount of information about the patient, the tumour and the treatment. The registries carefully collate all the data for any one patient to avoid duplication of records. This is not a quick process, as information is often not made available to the registry until the main course of treatment is finished. A sub-set of the data, as defined in the cancer registration minimum data set[7] is sent to the national registry at the ONS office in Titchfield, near Southampton. The data items are:

Core	Optional
Record type (new registration, amendment, deletion)	Country of birth
	Ethnic origin*
Identity number (unique)	Patient's occupation
Patient's name	Patient's employment status
Patient's previous surname	Patient's industry
Patient's address	Head of household's occupation
Postcode	Head of household's status
employment	Head of household's industry
Sex	Registration from screening*
NHS number	
Marital status	
Date of birth	
Date of death (if dead)	
Incidence date	
Site of primary growth	
Type of growth	
Behaviour of growth	
Multiple tumour indicator	
Basis of diagnosis*	
Death certificate only indicator*	
Side (laterality)*	
Treatment(s) (indicators)*	
Stage†	
Grade†	

* From incidence year 1993
† From incidence year 1993; phased introduction - initially only for breast and cervix.

The data are loaded onto the new person-based database (see below) and validated. The extensive checks include the compatibility of the cancer site and the associated histology; these checks are closely based on those promulgated by IARC[1]. Once all the expected records for any one incidence year have been received and validated at ONS, detailed tables are published on the numbers and rates of all types of cancer by age and sex, and by region of residence[8].

All the work on processing in Titchfield and flagging at the NHSCR in Southport has, since 1993, been paid for by the Department of Health (DH). A service level agreement (SLA) has been negotiated between DH and ONS. Work on the key targets and outputs established in the relevant ONS divisional business plans and the SLA is monitored continuously. ONS makes formal six-monthly progress reports to DH.

Redevelopment of the ONS cancer registration computer system

Beginning in 1990, over 20 of the major computer processing systems at the (then) OPCS - including births, deaths, cancer registrations, the Longitudinal Study (1% linked sample from the censuses), marriages and divorces - were redeveloped onto a modern database environment. The two main objectives of the redevelopment of the cancer registration computer system were to have an effective and efficient processing system; and a person-based database (rather than annual files of tumours). To meet the timetable for introducing the new system, it was necessary to convert the 21 annual tumour files (1971 to 1991 inclusive) to a person-based database before the new system began operation. From among the 4.5 million records, those which were either duplicates or were true multiple primary records for the same person were linked together by a probability matching process[9] based on those successfully operated by the Oxford Record Linkage Study, Statistics Canada, and the Information and Statistics Division (ISD) of the Scottish Health Service[10,11,12]. Information on linked registrations was sent to the cancer registries for the deletion or amendment of records as appropriate. The essential structure of the cancer registration system in England and Wales, shown in Figure A above has remained unchanged; but the identification, and the sending to the regional cancer registries, of the death certificates mentioning cancer and the non-cancer deaths to flagged cases, is now done by the new system in Titchfield. In addition, all validation errors are now returned to the appropriate registry for resolution.

In parallel with the work on the redevelopment of the system at ONS, a very large amount of data enhancement work was completed. This included 13,000 new registrations, amendments and cancellations; amendments to about 40,000 records from the probability matching exercise; 15,000 updates of date of death; 25,000 date of birth and date of death discrepancies; 7,000 no trace indicators added to the database; and smaller numbers of trace and event rejects, multiple primary cancer queries from registries, mis-traced Welsh records, "dead" now known to be alive, sex discrepancies, partial or invalid postcodes, and embarks. In addition, 36,000 queries from NHSCR about possible multiple primary cancers were dealt with.

The backlog of over 600,000 records which had built up in the registries during the time that the person-based database was being constructed was successfully processed by the NCIC in Titchfield. Priority for the processing of amendments resulting from validation errors was given to data for incidence years 1990 and 1991. At the same time, the NCIC worked steadily through the remaining problems - some left over from the old computer system, and some new ones. These included amendments to the way the system handled the notifications to the registries of death certificates containing a mention of cancer; corrections to records with duplicate identity numbers; re-numbering of some records for one regional registry; and improvements to postcodes. In addition, the revalidation - to the higher standards embedded in the new system - of all the data which had previously been processed on the old computer system has been carried out, queries sent to the regional registries and records amended. The new NHS numbers for flagged cases, together with any dates of death, were sent from the NHSCR to Titchfield, and passed to the cancer registries. This information has enabled both ONS and the registries to amend records for the "immortals" - cases registered alive but whose death was not previously linked to the cancer registration.

The backlog of records which had been processed in Titchfield was sent to the NHSCR in Southport once the testing of the module of their new computer system which deals with the flagging of cancer cases had been completed. It was known that about 65,000 of these were for people who had died before 1991 when the computerised index was assembled, and so they would not be on the database at NHSCR. These records were therefore stripped off the Titchfield database and sent separately to Southport on paper. Of the remaining records, which were sent on electronic media, it was expected that about 300,000 would match automatically on the system. It was planned to do the batch runs in order, ie the earliest registrations first, to facilitate the determination of true multiple cancers and duplicates. The flagging of the stockpiled registrations for incidence years 1971 to 1990 was completed in January 1997; and the resulting trace and event (death, embark, re-entry) data were sent to Titchfield and added to the database. All flagging for records up to incidence year 2002 which have been received at ONS and have passed the validation checks has been completed and work is in progress on cases diagnosed in 2003 and 2004. At the same time, ONS is attempting to keep earlier incidence years up to date by processing and flagging any "late" registrations received from the cancer registries.

Proposed extension to the cancer registration minimum data set

A conflict exists between the number of data items collected and data quality. This has been recognised by the three reviews of the national system described above[3,4,6]. The minimum data set has been revised in the context of the wider National Cancer Data Set and includes the stage of disease for all cancers, and details of treatment. This will require the information on stage to be made explicit by clinicians. Although the private sector is not covered by the minimum data set, members of the Independent Healthcare Association have generally been very co-operative; however, the growth of private pathology laboratories is a concern.

Processing problems

There have been three main problems with the cancer registration process. First, the timeliness of national data based on the full set of individual records depends on the speed of the slowest registry in completing its submissions to ONS. In the past, there has always been (at least) one registry which, for a variety of excellent reasons at the time, has lagged considerably behind the others. The most timely complete results were those for 1982 and 1983 which were published in 1985 and 1986 and were therefore only two years out of date. With the co-operation of the registries, however, it was possible to produce provisional results for 1990 to 1993 well in advance of the corresponding reference volumes.

Second, the database is "live" or "dynamic" in the sense that records may be modified or deleted if new information is obtained. The information from "trace back" of a death certificate may result in a case being registered many years after the true incidence date. This, together with the general timeliness problem, meant that any attempts in the past to bring forward the publication of national results has artefactually reduced the numbers of cases reported in the OPCS and ONS reference volumes. For several incidence years in the mid-1980s, there are now around 10% more cases on the national register than when the reference volumes were published (see Figure 1B in Appendix 1). Recently, however, several registries have redeveloped their computer systems (as has ONS) and their timeliness has improved dramatically. The availability of complete information for incidence years up to 1996 from half of the registries enabled ONS to produce in 1999 reliable provisional results for 1994 to 1996 for the 20 or so major cancer sites[13]. Less than a year later, similar provisional results up to 1997 were published[14].

Third, cancer registration is not statutory, and ONS has no organisational, managerial or financial control over the regional registries. In 1994, the registries passed from regional control to lead purchasers. Local needs for up to date information have in some areas resulted in considerable improvements in timeliness. On the other hand, although safeguards, and quality and timeliness standards, for national data were included in the national core contract[15,16], the requirements of lead purchasers who hold the registries' budgets sometimes took priority over the supply of data to ONS. In short, there was a power vacuum which, together with chronic underfunding of registries over a long period, means that it had been difficult to obtain timely, accurate and comparable data at the national level.

Advisory Committee on Cancer Registration review 1999/2000

In recent years, and particularly since the publication in 1995 of the Calman-Hine report on cancer services[17], the role of cancer registries has been extended. Cancer registries have contributed to studies on the variations in the outcomes for cancer patients across the UK and in the investigations into the underlying causes of these variations. Cancer registries were also increasingly being asked to provide data to support the planning and monitoring of cancer service delivery, including the national breast and cervical screening programmes. For these purposes, more extensive data sets are needed and the timeliness of information is of great importance. For the purposes of clinical governance, data on the patterns of care and outcomes for specified sub-groups of patients, for example defined by extent of disease or "stage", are needed.

This expansion of the traditional role of cancer registries led to renewed interest in them, but drew attention to the variable quality of the service that individual registries provided. Concerns were expressed about their capacity to provide up to date, complete and accurate data.

Despite the changes implemented following the three national reviews described above, these concerns had persisted, and in April 1999 the Advisory Committee on Cancer Registration, on behalf of the Department of Health, commissioned Professor Charles Gillis, then Director of the West of Scotland Cancer Surveillance Unit, to undertake a further review of cancer registration in England.

The review[18] found that due to the history of the cancer registries, which had grown up more or less autonomously since before the second world war, there were considerable variations among them in terms of organisational structures; type of host institution (hospital, health authority, academic); title; data collection process (predominantly manual or electronic); range of tumours registered; data items collected; IT systems; research activity; and significant variations in completeness, accuracy and timeliness of data submission to ONS. The budgets per head of population served and the cost per case registered appeared to vary considerably, although those for the majority of registries clustered closely around the average.

The timeliness of data acquisition by some of the registries had been poor, with the knock on effect that they were, in turn, slow in submitting data to ONS for national collation. For example, it was only in August 1997 that provisional figures were published for cancers diagnosed in 1992 - so at first sight national cancer registration data looked five years out of date - and confirmed registrations for 1991 were only published in December 1997. But as noted above, the timeliness of several registries improved dramatically during the late 1990s following redevelopment of their computer systems, and the provisional results up to incidence year 1996 were only two years out of date (and two years behind the available mortality data).

The issue of timeliness was addressed through the allocation by the Department of Health of £500,000 from the Public Health Development Fund, with the aim of ensuring a measurable improvement in the timeliness and quality of national cancer incidence and survival data. The target was that through this investment, all cancer registries would submit complete data up to and including 1997, to the quality standard in the national core contract, to ONS by the end of September 2000.

The review noted that data quality varied between registries. The editors of *Cancer Incidence in Five Continents Volume VII*[19] assess the quality of data submitted by individual cancer registries. It was a matter of concern that not all cancer registries in England provided data acceptable to the editors of this standard work.

Most cancer registries collect far more data than required for the national minimum data set. The review found tensions regarding the priority given to local and national need for data. In some cases, national priorities were unduly neglected. Some cancer registries had not complied with the requirement to submit data to ONS within the timescales specified in the national core contract. Data on variables relating to stage of disease and treatment were variably collected. Registries generally only collected information on treatment given within six months of diagnosis, as specified in the core contract, and so surgical, radiotherapy and chemotherapy treatments given later in the course of a patient's illness would have been excluded.

The review concluded that the credibility of the data for comparisons of the risks of cancer over time, and of outcomes within some cancer registry areas was well established. But the reliability of inter-regional comparisons was doubtful and the requirement for data of a uniform high standard in all parts of England, for the purposes of public health and clinical governance was certainly not being met.

The review made a number of key recommendations for how cancer registries should be strengthened, so that they would be able to contribute fully to the cancer modernisation agenda by providing robust data to support the planning and monitoring of cancer service delivery and identify the scope for NHS intervention in relation to deprivation and cancer. The Department of Health has published an action[20] plan to improve the organisation and effectiveness of the cancer registries in England. An additional £2 million of funding was allocated to cancer registration in each of the three financial years 2001/2 to 2003/4, a National Co-ordinator for Cancer Registration was appointed, and a National Cancer Registry Advisory Group was established.

References

1. Parkin DM, Chen VW, Ferlay J, Galceran J, Storm HH, Whelan SL. *Comparability and Quality Control in Cancer Registration*. IARC Technical Report No. 19. Lyons: International Agency for Research on Cancer, 1994.
2. Jensen OM, Parkin DM, Maclennan R, Muir CS, Skeet RG (eds). *Cancer Registration: Principles and Methods*. IARC Scientific Publications No.95. Lyons: International Agency for Research on Cancer, 1991.

3. Office of Population Censuses and Surveys. *Report of the Advisory Committee on Cancer Registration*. London: OPCS, 1970.
4. Office of Population Censuses and Surveys. *Report of the Advisory Committee on Cancer Registration, 1980: Cancer registration in the 1980s*. Series MB1 no.6. London: HMSO, 1981.
5. Department of Health. *Working for Patients. The Health Service. Caring for the 1990s*. CM 555. London: HMSO, 1989.
6. Office of Population Censuses and Surveys. *A Review of the National Cancer Registration System in England and Wales*. Series MB1 no.17. London: HMSO, 1990.
7. NHS Management Executive. *Minimum data set for the National Cancer Registration System*. EL(92)95. London: Department of Health, 1992.
8. Office for National Statistics. *Cancer statistics, - registrations, England 1998*. Series MB1 no.29. London: The Stationery Office, 2001.
9. Quinn MJ, Charlton JRH. Person-based follow-up of cancer cases: linkage using fuzzy matching. Proc Int Conf IASS/IAOS Satellite Meeting on Longitudinal Studies, Jerusalem, 1997.
10. Gill LE, Simmons HM. *An algorithm for fixed-length proper name compression: Oxford Name Compression Algorithm* (ONCA). University of Oxford, Unit of Clinical Epidemiology, 1992.
11. Newcombe HB. *Handbook of Record Linkage - Methods for Health and Statistical Studies, Administration and Business*. Oxford: Oxford Medical Publications, Oxford University Press, 1988.
12. Kendrick S, Clarke J. The Scottish Record Linkage System. Health Bulletin (Edinburgh) **51** No.2, March 1993.
13. Quinn MJ, Babb PJ, Jones J, Brock A. Report: Registrations of cancer diagnosed in 1993-1996, England and Wales. *Health Statistics Quarterly* 1999; **4**: 59-70.
14. Quinn MJ, Babb PJ, Kirby EA, Brock A. Report: Registrations of cancer diagnosed in 1994-1997, England and Wales. *Health Statistics Quarterly* 2000; **7**: 71-82.
15. NHS Executive. *Core contract for purchasing Cancer Registration*. EL(96)7. London: NHS Executive, 1996.
16. Winyard G. EL(96)7: *Core contract for purchasing cancer registration* (letter). Leeds: NHS Executive, 1998.
17. Department of Health and Welsh Office. *A policy framework for commissioning cancer services. A report by the Expert Advisory Group on Cancer to the Chief Medical Officers of England and Wales*. London: Department of Health, 1995. (Calman-Hine report.)
18. Cancer Registration in England: A way forward. [The "Gillis" Report.] Department of Health 2001: http://www.doh.gov.uk/cancer
19. Parkin DM, Whelan SL, Ferlay J, Raymond L, Young J. *Cancer Incidence in Five Continents, Volume VII*. IARC Scientific Publications No.143. Lyons: International Agency for Research on Cancer, 1997.
20. Action Programme for Cancer Registration. Department of Health 2001: http://www.doh.gov.uk/cancer

The United Kingdom Association of Cancer Registries

In the early 1990s, the cancer registration system in the UK was subject to rapid change. With the development of information technology, the pace of change in registration practice quickened, and increasing demands for accurate and timely information were made on the cancer registration system. Changes in the organisation of the health service and in the methods of health care delivery contributed to an increased interest from various authorities and scientists. There were new uses which could and should be made of registration data, such as medical audit and quality assurance of health care, as well as the routine uses which have been made of these data in the past, such as estimation of incidence and evaluation of survival and mortality.

There was widespread awareness both of the need to improve the quality and completeness of cancer registration data, and of the opportunities to do so through the use of information technology. Together with the increased interest from external bodies in using the data, this led to the creation of several groups bringing together cancer registry staff and personnel from OPCS (as it then was) to discuss and resolve matters of common interest.

The longest standing of these was the *Cancer Registries' Consultative Group* (CRCG) which concerns itself essentially with issues of data collection, including coding and data quality. It now has representation from all cancer registries in the UK and Ireland, and its members are for the most part registry managers and others closely involved in the day-to-day business of data collection. *The Cancer Surveillance Group* (CSG) was set up in 1989 to meet a perceived need for a forum bringing together those with an interest in the use of cancer data. It has a loose, open and informal membership and structure. Its members include epidemiologists and statisticians, as well as other registry staff. The *Cancer Registries' Information Technology Group* (CRITG) brings together technical experts from the various registries. Education and training was another area of activity thought to be of such importance that it could justify the establishment of another group. There was, however, no forum which brought together registry directors on a regular basis. There was a danger, therefore, with so many different perspectives and forums in which different points of view could be expressed, that the cancer registries might fail to speak with a united voice when, for example, making representations or giving advice to government. With no coherent framework of organisation, there would be a strong possibility of duplication of effort and inadequate communication between the various groups.

It was therefore proposed that a United Kingdom Association of Cancer Registries be established. Following preliminary meetings at which almost all of the UK registries were represented, the Association was brought into being on 2nd April 1992 in Cardiff.

The Association has a federal structure. All affiliated population-based cancer registries in the United Kingdom, ONS, the Information and Statistics Division of the NHS in Scotland and the Northern Ireland Cancer Registry are full members with their representative, usually the director, having a vote on the Executive Committee. Associate (non-voting) members currently (March 2002) comprise the National Registry of Ireland, the Childhood Cancer Research Group in Oxford, the CRC Paediatric and Familial Cancer Research Group in Manchester, the Northern Region Children and Young Persons Malignant Disease Registry in Newcastle, the West Midlands Regional Children's Tumour Registry in Birmingham, the Yorkshire Specialist Register of Cancer in Children and Young People in Leeds, and the charities Cancer Research UK and Marie Curie Cancer Care . Since the formation of the UKACR, a Quality Assurance group was set up to standardise the methodology for, and report on, various registry performance indicators included in the national core contract[1,2] such as timeliness and the percentage of registrations made solely from a death certificate. A Training Group and a Coding and Classification Group were established to oversee and co-ordinate the implementation of developments in those particular aspects of cancer registries' work. And a Clinical Effectiveness Group took forward issues relating to the registries' expanding role in clinical audit and performance monitoring on cancer. The Chairs of the various sub-groups, were invited, as appropriate, to attend Executive Committee meetings as observers.

In 2003, the structure of the UKACR's sub-groups was re-organised. Three new sub-groups were established, chaired by a registry director, and with new terms of reference and some decision making powers delegated from the Executive Committee. The Registration Sub-group has the former Coding and Classification Group and the Quality Assurance Group reporting to it. The other groups are the Information, Communications and Technology Sub-group, and the Analysis Sub-group.

The current (2003) officers are: Chair - Professor D Forman, Director of Information and Research at the Northern and Yorkshire Cancer Registry and Information Service; Vice Chair - Dr D Brewster, Director of the Scottish Cancer Registry; and

Treasurer - Mrs S Reynolds, of the Welsh Cancer Intelligence and Surveillance Unit. It was agreed that ONS was the most appropriate body to provide secretariat facilities; Dr M J Quinn (Director of the NCIC) was nominated by ONS to be the Association's Executive Secretary.

The UKACR provides:
- a focus for national initiatives in cancer registration;
- a coherent voice for representation of cancer registries in the United Kingdom;
- a channel for liaison between registries and for agreeing policy on matters connected with cancer registration;
- a framework to facilitate the operation of special interest groups and regional registries;
  and
- a means of stimulating the development of cancer registration, of information procedures and practices, and of research based on cancer registry data.

The UKACR represents the views of its members to government and other bodies operating at national level on issues concerned with data quality, the definition of information requirements, and the development of health information systems where these have implications for cancer registration, in particular where matters of overall policy are concerned. The Association was represented on the re-formed National Advisory Committee on Cancer Registration and currently on the Cancer Registration Advisory Group (CRAG). The establishment of such close links is very important given the intimate ties many regional registries have with NHS information systems, and the potential importance of cancer registration to NHS functions such as medical audit and contracting.

The UKACR has, through consensus, examined and improved coding and classification issues; agreed the complex interface document for transmission of data to and from ONS; developed performance indicators; produced a training manual and cancer-specific training packs for registry staff; developed guidelines for the release of data, including for the rapidly expanding field of genetic counselling; developed guidelines for standardisation of reported results; and established a forum for sharing the latest epidemiological research. Consensus may be slower to achieve than coercion, but may in practice be stronger and more valuable as there is often a better chance that an agreed procedure will actually be followed. Even near consensus requires those disagreeing to continually justify their minority position.

References

1. NHS Executive. *Core contract for purchasing Cancer Registration*. EL(96)7. London: NHS Executive, 1996.
2. Winyard G. EL(96)7: *Core contract for purchasing cancer registration* (letter). Leeds: NHS Executive, 1998.

Cancer registrations, 2001

Interpretation

Care is required in the interpretation of cancer registration statistics, particularly when addressing either trends over time or differences between regions.

Registration of cases of cancer is a dynamic process in the sense that the data files both in the cancer registries and at ONS are always open. Cancer records may be amended - for example, the site code may be modified should later, more accurate, information become available. The date of death is added for cases registered when the person was alive. Records may be cancelled, although this is relatively unusual. Also, complete new 'late' registrations may be made after either the cancer registry, or ONS, or both, have published what were thought at the time to be virtually complete results for a particular year.

Consequently, the figures for registrations published by a cancer registry in its reference volume may be different from those in the corresponding annual reference volume published by ONS in the series MB1, which will generally have been produced at a different (usually later) time. In addition, both sets of published figures will differ again from the numbers of registrations currently on the databases. Further differences between cancer registry and ONS figures may arise if records which have been rejected by the validation process at ONS have not been corrected by the registry concerned before the corresponding ARV tables are produced.

In the section on 'Validity' in Appendix 1, it is noted that the cancer registries probably differ in their levels of completeness of registration. It may be difficult to interpret any apparent trends in cancer registrations because the registries are continually striving to increase their levels of ascertainment of cases. Any particularly large increases from year to year in the numbers of registrations for an individual registry are most likely to have arisen because of this.

Other aspects of the cancer registration system which are relevant to the interpretation of the data include: geographic coverage; methods of data collection; ascertainment (or completeness of registration); completeness of recording of data items; validity; accuracy; late registrations, deletions and amendments; duplicate and multiple registrations; registrations from information on death certificates; clinical and pathological definitions and diagnoses; changes in coding systems; completeness of flagging at NHSCR; changes in definition of resident population; and error. These are discussed in detail in Appendix 1.

ONS has been advised both by expert epidemiologists and by members of the former Steering Committee on Cancer Registration, that non-melanoma skin cancer (ICD10 C44) is greatly under-registered. Registration varies widely depending on a registry's degree of access to out-patient records and general practitioners. This under-registration of non-melanoma skin cancer is not just a problem for the cancer registries in England. *Cancer Incidence in Five Continents Volume VI*[1] reported that cancer registries in the United States, Australia, and parts of Europe, also collected a very limited information on these skin cancers. In the commentary which follows, the figures for 'all malignancies' **exclude non-melanoma skin cancer** (nmsc).

Cancer registrations in England, 2001

In 2001 there were totals of around 151,000 registrations of cases of cancer for males and 170,000 for females. In the 10th revision of the International Statistical Classification of Diseases and Related Health Problems (ICD10), malignant neoplasms are coded C00-C97 and benign, in situ, uncertain and unspecified neoplasms are coded D00-D48. In 2001, of the total registrations about 11,700 for males and 34,500 for females were non-malignant. Around two thirds of the non-malignant neoplasms for females were carcinoma in situ of the cervix (ICD10 D06).

Cancer is predominantly a disease of the elderly. The overall crude rates of cancer registrations (excluding nmsc), 466 per 100,000 population for males and 444 per 100,000 population for females, conceal wide differences between the sexes and across the age groups, as illustrated in Figure B. The numbers on which this Figure is based are given in Table 3. Following the small decrease in rates after early childhood, rates increased continuously across the age range for both males and females. A falling off in the rates for the very elderly (85 years and over) may indicate under-registration; this does not seem to have occurred. Rates of cancer rose more quickly with age in females than in males; this is reflected in the age distribution described below. In the 40–44 age group, the rate in females was double that for males. Subsequently, the overall rates rose more rapidly for males and were broadly similar to those for females in the 55–59 age group. After this, the rates rose much more rapidly for males - they were almost 50 per cent higher than those for females in the 65–69 age group and almost double in those aged 80–84.

The age distribution of malignant neoplasms is shown in Figure C. The numbers on which this Figure is based are given in Table 1.

Of the total of 224,650 registrations, only 1,170 (0.5 per cent) occurred in children aged under 15; of these, 365 (31 per cent) were leukaemias (ICD10 C91-C95). The percentages of cancers in the five-year age-groups tended to rise earlier in females than in males, owing largely to the influence of the incidence of cancers of the breast (ICD10 C50) and of the cervix (ICD10 C53). Cancers in those aged under 45 amounted to just over 5 per cent of the total for males and just under 9 per cent for females. The peaks in the age distributions occurred in the 70–79 age groups for males, and the 75–79 age group for females.

The standardised registration ratios by GOR are illustrated in Figure D. The numbers on which this figure is based are given in Table 6. These SRRs should be interpreted with caution because it is difficult to separate the effect of variation in levels of ascertainment from genuine differences in incidence.

Major cancer sites

In the ICD 10th Revision, there are 88 3-digit site codes relating to malignant neoplasms; of these, four relate to males only and eight to females only. For both males and females just **three** of the sites (different ones for each sex) constituted just over half of the total registrations in 2001, as shown in Table A.

The numbers of registrations for the major sites are illustrated in Figure E (and given in Table 1). The numbers of registrations for the 17 sites (counting lip and mouth, colorectal, non-Hodgkin's lymphoma and leukaemia each as one) for males represent 89 per cent of the total; those for the 19 sites for females represent 88 per cent.

Figure B   All malignant neoplasms (excluding C44): incidence rates by age group, 2001

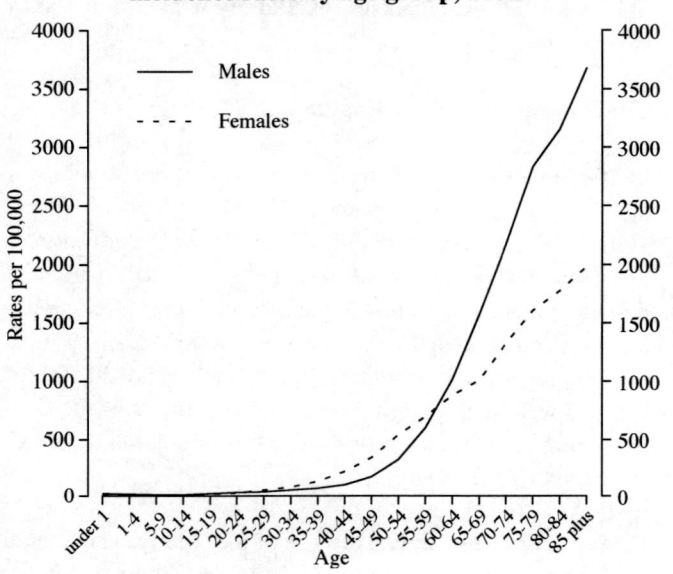

Figure C   All malignant neoplasms (excluding nmsc): frequency distribution by age group, 2001

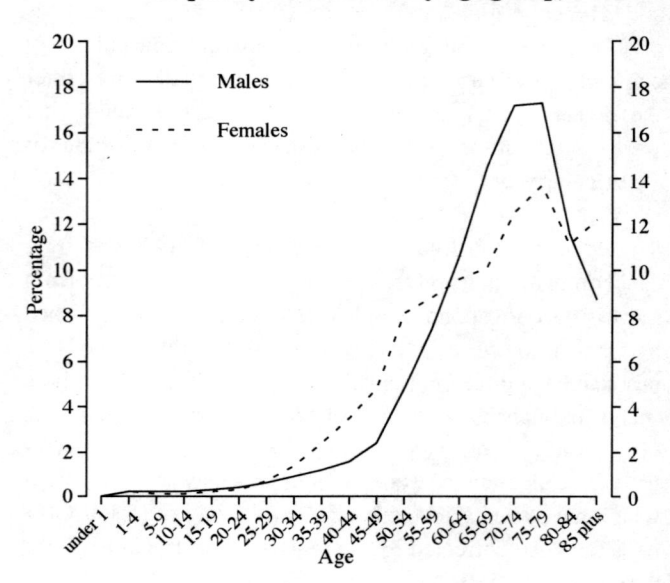

Table A   The three most common cancers, 2001

	ICD10	Site description	Number of registrations	% of total malignancies
(a)	Males			
1	C61	Prostate	26,027	23.1
2	C34	Lung	18,545	16.5
3	C18-20	Colorectal	14,836	13.2
		Total	59,408	52.8
		All malignancies*	112,516	100
(b)	Females			
1	C50	Breast	34,347	30.6
2	C18-20	Colorectal	12,693	11.3
3	C34	Lung	11,940	10.6
		Total	58,980	52.6
		All malignancies*	112,134	100

Reference

1. Parkin DM, Muir CS, Whelan SL, Gao Y-T, Ferlay J, Powell J. *Cancer Incidence in Five Continents. Volume VI.* IARC Scientific Publications No. 120. Lyons: International Agency for Research on Cancer, 1993.

Figure D All malignant neoplasms (excluding C44): standardised registration ratios by GOR, 2001

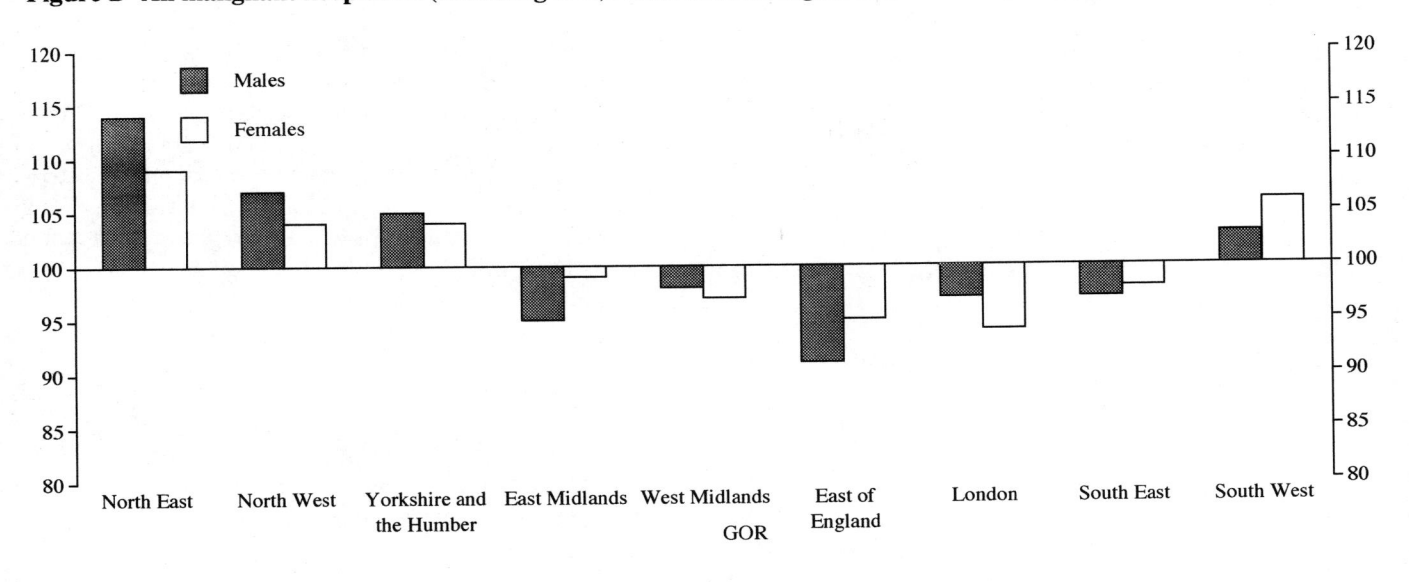

Figure E Registrations - major sites, 2001

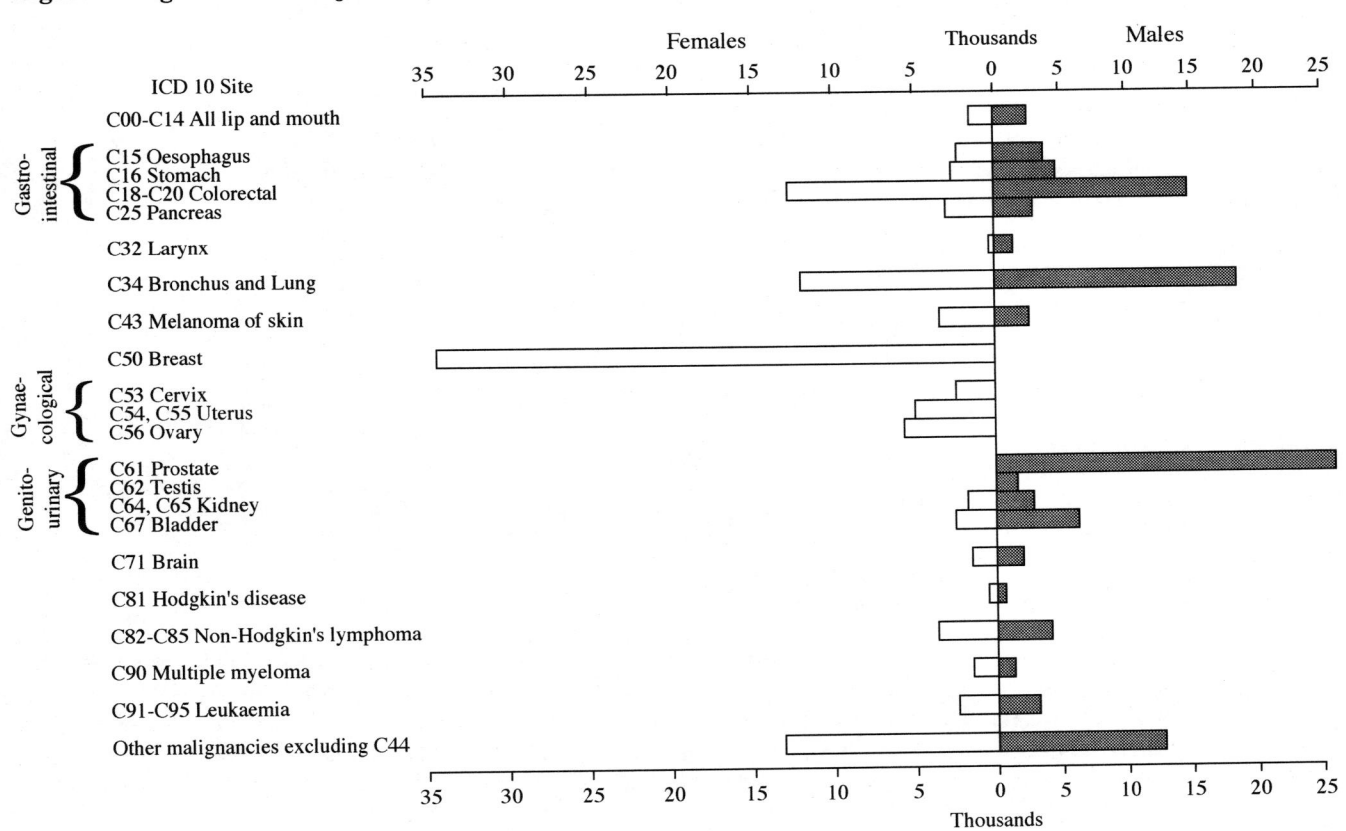

Cumulative risk of cancer

The cumulative risk of a person being registered with a malignant cancer (ICD-10 sites C00-C97 excluding C44) can be estimated[1], for males and females separately, by applying sex- and age-specific cancer registration rates to the person years at risk derived from the numbers of survivors from a cohort based on an England life table. Such a cohort is hypothetical, not a birth cohort, being entirely dependent on the age-specific death rates prevailing in the year for which it was constructed.

For example, for males aged 65 there would be 77,261 person years at risk in 2001. The cancer registration rate for all malignant neoplasms (excluding ICD-10 C44) in 2001 for this age was 1,369 per 100,000. Thus one would expect there to be

$$77,261 \times 1,369 \div 100,000 = 1,058 \text{ registrations}$$

or 1.1 per cent of the original cohort.

The detailed calculations are carried out for each single year of age. The corresponding percentages for five year age groups, and the cumulative percentages of risk are illustrated in Figure F. It can be seen that 39 per cent of the cohort of males and 35 per cent of the female cohort would eventually be registered with some form of malignancy. However, registrations would not be equally spread across age-groups. Only 7 per cent of the cohort of males (one sixth of the total) and 10 per cent of the cohort of females (just over one quarter of the total) would be registered at ages below 60.

Reference

1 Schouten LJ, Straatman H, Kiemeney LALM & Verbeek ALM. Cancer incidence: life table risk versus cumulative risk. Journal of Epidemiology and Community Health 1994; 48: 596-600.

Figure F Cumulative risk of incidence of all neoplasms by age and sex, England, 2001

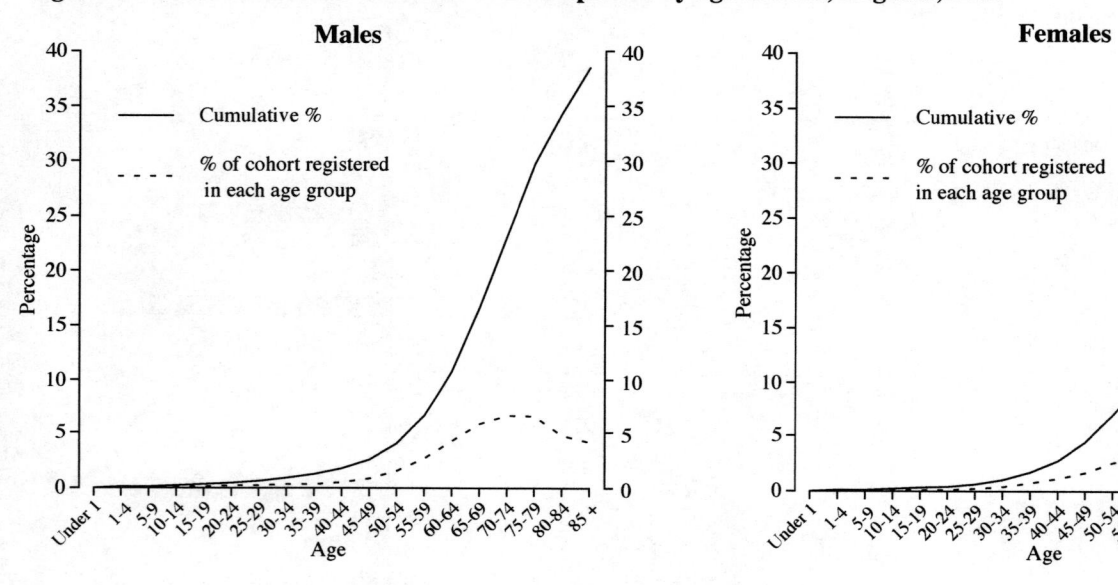

Cancer incidence in the UK, 1999–2001

Table B gives the three-year averages for registrations of newly diagnosed cases and directly age-standardised rates (using the European standard population) for selected cancers during 1999-2001, for the UK and its four constituent countries. The table has been compiled with assistance from the cancer registries in Wales, Scotland and Northern Ireland.

In 1999-2001, there was an average of around 133,700 registrations per year for males and 135,900 for females in the UK. The corresponding overall registration rates were just over 400 and 340 per 100,000 population for males and females, respectively.

The incidence of breast cancer in females was higher than of lung cancer for males and females combined in the UK as a whole, and in each of England, Wales and Northern Ireland. In Scotland however, the incidence of breast cancer was only four fifths of total lung cancer incidence.

The incidence of prostate cancer was higher than that of lung cancer in males in the UK as a whole, as well as in England and in Wales. In Scotland however, the incidence of lung cancer was just over 30% higher than that of prostate cancer. Colorectal cancer was the third most common cancer among males.

Breast cancer had the highest incidence of all cancers in females in the UK as a whole, and in each of the constituent countries. Colorectal and lung cancers were the second and third most common, respectively, except in Scotland where the incidence of lung cancer was 14% higher than that of colorectal cancer.

In Scotland, the incidence of lung cancer in both males and females was much higher than that in England, Wales and Northern Ireland. The incidence of cancers of the lip, mouth and pharynx, oesophagus, and larynx was also particularly high in Scotland compared with the other countries.

Table B Registrations and directly age standardised[1] registration rates per 100,000 population of newly diagnosed cases of cancer: selected sites by sex and country, United Kingdom, 1999-2001[2]

ICD10	Site description	Sex	United Kingdom Number	Rate	England Number	Rate	Wales Number	Rate	Scotland[3] Number	Rate	N Ireland Number	Rate
C00-C97 x C44	All malignancies excluding nmsc[3]	M	133,697	403.4	110,972	398.6	7,738	437.8	11,878	431.2	3,110	392.1
		F	135,934	343.0	112,134	339.1	7,480	357.6	12,954	370.1	3,367	345.0
C00-C14	Lip, mouth & pharynx	M	3,277	10.7	2,582	10.0	186	11.6	422	16.1	87	11.4
		F	1,832	4.8	1,467	4.6	107	5.3	209	6.3	48	5.0
C15	Oesophagus	M	4,493	13.7	3,682	13.3	263	15.0	459	16.7	90	11.5
		F	2,864	5.9	2,321	5.7	172	6.9	305	7.3	66	5.9
C16	Stomach	M	6,049	17.9	4,962	17.5	391	21.7	545	19.6	150	18.7
		F	3,454	7.1	2,740	6.7	231	8.7	381	9.0	102	8.8
C18-C20	Colorectal	M	18,442	55.3	15,069	53.8	1,103	62.0	1,795	64.8	476	60.2
		F	15,939	35.2	13,004	34.4	888	36.6	1,617	41.0	430	40.1
C25	Pancreas	M	3,367	10.2	2,828	10.2	191	10.9	273	10.0	75	9.6
		F	3,637	7.7	3,039	7.7	212	8.2	315	7.7	71	6.3
C32	Larynx	M	1,920	6.1	1,502	5.7	110	6.5	252	9.5	56	7.3
C34	Lung	M	23,130	68.7	18,932	66.9	1,203	66.2	2,462	88.1	532	66.9
		F	14,878	35.0	11,929	33.6	763	34.1	1,847	49.2	340	33.8
C43	Melanoma of skin	M	2,931	9.4	2,447	9.4	134	8.3	273	10.3	77	9.8
		F	3,833	10.9	3,195	11.0	155	8.4	365	11.7	118	12.7
C50	Breast	F	40,740	114.6	34,100	115.0	2,121	113.4	3,574	114.6	945	106.0
C53	Cervix	F	3,045	9.1	2,495	8.9	162	9.7	304	10.4	83	9.6
C54	Uterus	F	5,490	14.9	4,569	14.8	335	17.3	451	14.1	135	15.0
C56	Ovary	F	6,663	18.0	5,490	17.8	403	20.5	594	18.0	176	19.7
C61	Prostate	M	27,362	79.8	23,329	81.1	1,642	88.3	1,873	66.1	518	64.6
C62	Testis	M	1,997	6.8	1,659	6.7	77	5.6	203	8.1	58	7.0
C64	Kidney	M	3,281	10.3	2,664	9.9	215	12.8	319	11.9	83	10.7
		F	2,057	5.2	1,658	5.0	125	6.0	218	6.1	56	5.8
C67	Bladder	M	8,101	23.9	6,786	23.8	646	35.9	525	18.8	143	17.9
		F	3,302	6.9	2,740	6.8	254	10.7	247	5.9	61	5.3
C71	Brain	M	2,467	8.1	2,049	8.0	146	9.2	209	8.1	63	8.0
		F	1,826	5.2	1,519	5.2	105	5.9	159	5.1	42	4.7
C81-C96	Lymphomas and Leukaemias	M	11,473	35.9	9,603	35.8	617	36.8	959	35.8	294	37.0
		F	9,681	24.1	8,036	24.0	519	24.8	869	24.6	257	25.2
C81-C85	Lymphomas	M	5,619	17.9	4,760	18.1	259	16.0	451	17.0	150	18.8
		F	4,948	12.9	4,093	12.8	243	12.2	461	13.6	151	15.4
C81	Hodgkin's disease	M	823	2.8	689	2.8	46	3.2	63	2.5	26	3.1
		F	607	2.0	505	2.0	29	1.9	57	2.1	16	1.9
C82-C85	Non-Hodgkin's lymphoma	M	4,796	15.1	4,071	15.2	212	12.9	389	14.4	124	15.7
		F	4,341	11.0	3,588	10.9	213	10.4	404	11.5	135	13.6
C90	Multiple myeloma	M	1,859	5.6	1,539	5.5	110	6.1	156	5.6	55	7.0
		F	1,688	3.8	1,403	3.8	94	4.0	143	3.6	47	4.3
C91-C95	Leukaemia	M	3,815	11.9	3,156	11.7	235	13.9	337	12.7	87	10.9
		F	2,921	7.1	2,438	7.1	176	8.3	251	7.1	56	5.3

1 Using the European standard population
2 Three-year averages
3 nmsc: non-melanoma skin cancer (C44)

Table 1 Series MB1 no. 32

Table 1 Registrations of newly diagnosed cases of cancer: site, sex and age, 2001

ICD (10th Revision) number	Site description		All ages	Age group								
				Under 1	1-4	5-9	10-14	15-19	20-24	25-29	30-34	35-39
	All registrations	M	151,069	70	220	189	212	326	519	804	1,294	1,796
		F	170,127	51	203	159	203	532	3,967	6,301	6,611	6,274
C00-C97	All cancers	M	139,387	56	214	176	189	294	465	715	1,170	1,604
		F	135,657	48	192	144	167	225	388	932	1,727	3,020
C00-C97 xC44	All cancers excluding nmsc	M	112,516	56	214	171	184	282	449	651	1,004	1,301
		F	112,134	47	192	143	163	211	360	840	1,552	2,636
C00-C14	Malignant neoplasm of lip, mouth and pharynx	M	2,606	1	-	2	4	6	9	17	22	47
		F	1,461	-	-	3	2	6	7	15	18	30
C00	Malignant neoplasm of lip	M	159	-	-	-	-	-	-	-	3	4
		F	79	-	-	-	-	-	1	-	-	-
C01	Malignant neoplasm of base of tongue	M	184	-	-	-	-	-	-	-	-	1
		F	63	-	-	-	-	-	-	-	-	-
C02	Malignant neoplasm of other and unspecified parts of tongue	M	443	-	-	-	-	1	3	6	10	11
		F	301	-	-	-	-	-	-	1	4	8	8
C03	Malignant neoplasm of gum	M	106	1	-	-	-	1	-	-	1	4
		F	88	-	-	-	-	1	-	-	-	-
C04	Malignant neoplasm of floor of mouth	M	241	-	-	-	-	-	-	-	1	2
		F	106	-	-	-	-	-	-	-	1	1
C05	Malignant neoplasm of palate	M	119	-	-	1	-	-	-	-	1	2
		F	104	-	-	-	-	-	1	3	4	2
C06	Malignant neoplasm of other and unspecified parts of mouth	M	199	-	-	-	-	-	1	1	-	3
		F	149	-	-	-	-	-	-	1	-	-
C07	Malignant neoplasm of parotid gland	M	199	-	-	-	1	1	-	4	4	5
		F	145	-	-	1	1	2	2	5	1	10
C08	Malignant neoplasm of other and unspecified major salivary glands	M	55	-	-	-	1	1	2	1	-	4
		F	50	-	-	1	1	-	-	-	-	3
C09	Malignant neoplasm of tonsil	M	332	-	-	-	-	-	-	-	1	6
		F	117	-	-	-	-	-	-	-	-	1
C10	Malignant neoplasm of oropharynx	M	104	-	-	-	-	-	-	-	-	-
		F	29	-	-	-	-	-	-	-	1	-
C11	Malignant neoplasm of nasopharynx	M	107	-	-	1	2	2	3	3	1	3
		F	64	-	-	-	-	3	2	2	2	4
C12	Malignant neoplasm of piriform sinus	M	165	-	-	-	-	-	-	1	-	-
		F	36	-	-	-	-	-	-	-	-	-
C13	Malignant neoplasm of hypopharynx	M	78	-	-	-	-	-	-	-	-	-
		F	69	-	-	-	-	-	-	-	1	-
C14	Malignant neoplasm of other and ill-defined sites in the lip, oral cavity and pharynx	M	115	-	-	-	-	-	-	1	-	2
		F	61	-	-	1	-	-	-	-	-	1
C15	Malignant neoplasm of oesophagus	M	3,806	-	-	-	-	1	-	2	8	16
		F	2,274	-	-	-	-	-	-	-	5	10
C16	Malignant neoplasm of stomach	M	4,741	1	-	-	-	1	1	5	20	18
		F	2,626	-	-	-	-	-	1	4	7	21
C17	Malignant neoplasm of small intestine	M	316	-	-	-	-	-	-	3	3	5
		F	275	-	-	-	-	-	1	-	2	4
C18-C20	Malignant neoplasm of colon and rectum	M	14,836	-	-	1	1	2	16	12	36	97
		F	12,693	-	-	-	5	6	8	15	47	70
C18	Malignant neoplasm of colon	M	8,858	-	-	1	1	1	11	9	26	56
		F	8,677	-	-	-	5	5	5	11	27	43
C19	Malignant neoplasm of rectosigmoid junction	M	1,205	-	-	-	-	-	1	1	1	4
		F	846	-	-	-	-	-	-	1	-	7

England
Registered by May 2004

40-44	45-49	50-54	55-59	60-64	65-69	70-74	75-79	80-84	85 and over	M/F	Site description	ICD (10th Revision) number
2,551	3,815	7,493	11,245	15,770	21,474	25,372	26,133	17,989	13,797	M	All registrations	
6,403	7,707	12,394	13,024	14,243	15,241	18,826	20,774	17,444	19,770	F		
2,298	3,458	6,904	10,363	14,617	19,920	23,482	24,138	16,569	12,755	M	All cancers	C00-C97
4,494	6,286	10,512	11,479	12,653	13,732	17,075	18,875	15,808	17,900	F		
1,757	2,711	5,445	8,352	11,960	16,296	19,318	19,483	13,062	9,820	M	All cancers excluding nmsc	C00-C97 xC44
3,911	5,437	9,132	9,869	10,721	11,370	14,046	15,311	12,480	13,713	F		
107	193	345	403	356	314	270	266	153	91	M	Malignant neoplasm of lip, mouth and pharynx	C00-C14
77	91	140	147	162	134	177	165	115	172	F		
6	9	12	11	17	14	25	29	16	13	M	Malignant neoplasm of lip	C00
2	3	1	4	7	10	9	11	10	21	F		
6	20	33	35	31	20	15	10	8	5	M	Malignant neoplasm of base of tongue	C01
3	9	8	13	5	5	7	8	4	1	F		
19	31	59	57	61	60	49	43	22	11	M	Malignant neoplasm of other and unspecified parts of tongue	C02
15	16	36	28	34	30	29	35	18	39	F		
8	9	9	14	12	8	7	15	9	8	M	Malignant neoplasm of gum	C03
2	3	2	9	11	11	14	16	6	13	F		
12	16	42	50	38	38	17	17	6	2	M	Malignant neoplasm of floor of mouth	C04
3	9	15	9	13	10	12	13	10	10	F		
4	6	16	28	17	12	10	9	7	6	M	Malignant neoplasm of palate	C05
9	10	9	9	9	3	17	14	7	7	F		
4	10	20	30	34	24	21	22	15	14	M	Malignant neoplasm of other and unspecified parts of mouth	C06
6	7	9	10	17	14	18	18	18	31	F		
8	11	16	16	13	16	24	37	30	13	M	Malignant neoplasm of parotid gland	C07
11	4	10	8	18	11	20	14	8	19	F		
2	-	5	6	5	12	4	7	3	2	M	Malignant neoplasm of other and unspecified major salivary glands	C08
3	3	3	7	2	4	7	6	4	6	F		
26	49	59	63	41	28	29	21	5	4	M	Malignant neoplasm of tonsil	C09
10	8	19	18	18	13	10	8	8	4	F		
2	5	16	22	14	15	13	8	7	2	M	Malignant neoplasm of oropharynx	C10
2	3	4	2	4	3	3	3	2	2	F		
5	9	18	14	14	10	9	6	6	1	M	Malignant neoplasm of nasopharynx	C11
7	7	9	8	7	1	2	4	2	4	F		
-	5	22	28	30	30	23	18	6	2	M	Malignant neoplasm of piriform sinus	C12
2	4	5	7	5	3	5	1	2	2	F		
3	5	8	10	11	10	13	8	5	5	M	Malignant neoplasm of hypopharynx	C13
2	3	3	9	7	7	17	5	10	5	F		
2	8	10	19	18	17	11	16	8	3	M	Malignant neoplasm of other and ill-defined sites in the lip, oral cavity and pharynx	C14
-	2	7	6	5	9	7	9	6	8	F		
47	114	249	360	470	512	656	629	457	285	M	Malignant neoplasm of oesophagus	C15
11	45	90	107	173	197	309	420	375	532	F		
61	95	188	296	446	616	897	897	679	520	M	Malignant neoplasm of stomach	C16
38	52	79	95	171	263	401	469	480	545	F		
8	11	23	34	38	49	47	50	22	23	M	Malignant neoplasm of small intestine	C17
11	7	11	24	33	33	35	41	35	38	F		
183	298	739	1,158	1,584	2,204	2,648	2,685	1,861	1,311	M	Malignant neoplasm of colon and rectum	C18-C20
163	290	541	793	1,044	1,398	1,878	2,258	1,917	2,260	F		
94	149	402	575	893	1,274	1,595	1,707	1,212	852	M	Malignant neoplasm of colon	C18
102	206	329	509	686	940	1,298	1,567	1,333	1,611	F		
12	35	52	113	147	192	231	211	125	80	M	Malignant neoplasm of rectosigmoid junction	C19
12	19	44	63	82	113	122	157	111	115	F		

Table 1 Series MB1 no. 32

Table 1   Registrations - *continued*

ICD (10th Revision) number	Site description		All ages	Under 1	1-4	5-9	10-14	15-19	20-24	25-29	30-34	35-39
C20	Malignant neoplasm of rectum	M F	4,773 3,170	- -	- -	- -	- -	1 1	4 3	2 3	9 20	37 20
C21	Malignant neoplasm of anus and anal canal	M F	255 385	- -	- -	- -	- -	- -	- 1	- 2	3 3	1 8
C22	Malignant neoplasm of liver and intrahepatic bile ducts	M F	1,242 883	6 3	6 4	- -	1 -	1 3	1 -	9 3	9 2	9 7
C23	Malignant neoplasm of gallbladder	M F	124 287	- -	- -	- -	- -	- -	- -	- -	- -	2 1
C24	Malignant neoplasm of other and unspecified parts of biliary tract	M F	291 307	- -	- 1	- -	- -	- -	- 1	- -	1 2	- 1
C25	Malignant neoplasm of pancreas	M F	2,807 2,986	- -	- -	- -	- -	- 1	- 1	2 -	5 4	27 10
C26	Malignant neoplasm of other and ill-defined digestive organs	M F	230 327	- -	- -	- 1	- -	- -	- -	1 -	- 1	4 2
C30	Malignant neoplasm of nasal cavity and middle ear	M F	100 88	- -	- -	1 -	- -	- 1	3 -	- -	2 3	4 3
C31	Malignant neoplasm of accessory sinuses	M F	90 54	- -	1 1	- -	- -	1 -	- 1	- 1	4 1	1 1
C32	Malignant neoplasm of larynx	M F	1,477 328	- -	- -	- -	- -	- -	- 1	3 -	3 1	9 2
C33-C34	Malignant neoplasm of trachea, bronchus and lung	M F	18,577 11,963	1 -	- 1	- -	- 1	3 1	2 1	8 6	21 21	48 40
C33	Malignant neoplasm of trachea	M F	32 23	- -	- -	- -	- -	- -	- -	- -	- -	- 1
C34	Malignant neoplasm of bronchus and lung	M F	18,545 11,940	1 -	- 1	- -	- 1	3 1	2 1	8 6	21 21	48 39
C37	Malignant neoplasm of thymus	M F	30 30	- -	- -	- -	- -	- -	- -	- 1	1 -	3 -
C38	Malignant neoplasm of heart, mediastinum and pleura	M F	136 97	2 -	2 1	- -	1 -	1 -	- -	5 -	4 1	1 2
C39	Malignant neoplasm of other and ill-defined sites in the respiratory system and intrathoracic organs	M F	4 3	- -	- -	- -	- -	- -	- -	- -	- -	- -
C40	Malignant neoplasm of bone and articular cartilage of limbs	M F	112 90	- -	1 -	7 4	18 8	17 15	5 4	7 3	6 5	3 4
C41	Malignant neoplasm of bone and articular cartilage of other and unspecified sites	M F	111 117	- -	1 2	2 3	4 4	7 5	7 5	5 4	7 5	4 7
C43	Malignant melanoma of skin	M F	2,638 3,424	- -	- -	- -	2 2	9 19	37 79	64 146	120 185	131 246
C44	Other malignant neoplasms of skin	M F	26,871 23,523	- 1	- -	5 1	5 4	12 14	16 28	64 92	166 175	303 384
C45	Mesothelioma	M F	1,423 329	- -	- -	- -	- -	- -	- -	1 -	- 2	1 2
C46	Kaposi's sarcoma	M F	63 17	- -	- -	- 1	- -	- -	2 -	2 -	14 4	10 3
C47	Malignant neoplasm of peripheral nerves and autonomic nervous system	M F	39 48	- -	4 5	2 1	2 -	1 1	- 1	1 5	1 2	2 3
C48	Malignant neoplasm of retroperitoneum and peritoneum	M F	97 183	- -	1 -	1 -	- -	1 -	- -	1 -	2 1	1 6

40-44	45-49	50-54	55-59	60-64	65-69	70-74	75-79	80-84	85 and over		Site description	ICD (10th Revision) number
77	114	285	470	544	738	822	767	524	379	M	Malignant neoplasm of rectum	C20
49	65	168	221	276	345	458	534	473	534	F		
12	11	26	37	27	33	35	30	22	18	M	Malignant neoplasm of anus and anal canal	C21
15	27	34	26	40	33	54	50	47	45	F		
25	44	81	108	144	161	194	212	121	110	M	Malignant neoplasm of liver and intrahepatic bile ducts	C22
13	8	31	45	66	93	135	180	153	137	F		
1	2	7	10	14	23	12	26	14	13	M	Malignant neoplasm of gallbladder	C23
6	5	12	29	12	39	46	49	34	54	F		
4	5	9	30	31	36	46	56	38	35	M	Malignant neoplasm of other and unspecified parts of biliary tract	C24
7	2	10	17	31	21	47	49	54	64	F		
37	85	133	209	316	426	457	474	328	308	M	Malignant neoplasm of pancreas	C25
36	39	101	157	229	297	439	522	544	606	F		
3	3	12	14	13	25	50	26	38	41	M	Malignant neoplasm of other and ill-defined digestive organs	C26
4	8	8	11	13	29	28	39	56	127	F		
4	5	10	11	8	13	14	10	5	10	M	Malignant neoplasm of nasal cavity and middle ear	C30
3	5	6	8	3	13	13	15	7	8	F		
2	6	8	12	7	10	12	13	9	4	M	Malignant neoplasm of accessory sinuses	C31
1	5	7	4	2	2	5	7	8	8	F		
20	54	149	211	215	249	227	170	101	66	M	Malignant neoplasm of larynx	C32
6	15	30	36	42	48	49	38	26	34	F		
122	339	764	1,344	2,031	2,789	3,586	3,688	2,319	1,512	M	Malignant neoplasm of trachea, bronchus and lung	C33-C34
106	273	609	838	1,157	1,476	2,251	2,358	1,644	1,180	F		
-	2	2	-	3	2	7	9	5	2	M	Malignant neoplasm of trachea	C33
-	1	2	3	3	-	6	4	1	2	F		
122	337	762	1,344	2,028	2,787	3,579	3,679	2,314	1,510	M	Malignant neoplasm of bronchus and lung	C34
106	272	607	835	1,154	1,476	2,245	2,354	1,643	1,178	F		
1	1	5	2	5	5	2	2	-	3	M	Malignant neoplasm of thymus	C37
4	2	9	1	1	4	4	2	2	-	F		
4	3	9	10	12	11	26	13	19	13	M	Malignant neoplasm of heart, mediastinum and pleura	C38
2	3	7	9	7	7	16	19	13	10	F		
-	-	-	-	-	2	1	-	-	1	M	Malignant neoplasm of other and ill-defined sites in the respiratory system and intrathoracic organs	C39
-	-	1	1	-	-	1	-	-	-	F		
6	8	5	6	3	3	1	8	5	3	M	Malignant neoplasm of bone and articular cartilage of limbs	C40
2	2	8	5	5	2	4	6	3	10	F		
6	3	3	11	11	9	7	10	9	5	M	Malignant neoplasm of bone and articular cartilage of other and unspecified sites	C41
5	-	8	7	6	9	12	11	9	15	F		
168	211	261	259	284	286	260	237	176	133	M	Malignant melanoma of skin	C43
265	295	336	316	240	285	282	273	248	207	F		
541	747	1,459	2,011	2,657	3,624	4,164	4,655	3,507	2,935	M	Other malignant neoplasms of skin	C44
583	849	1,380	1,610	1,932	2,362	3,029	3,564	3,328	4,187	F		
4	23	68	139	210	245	244	279	135	74	M	Mesothelioma	C45
2	11	14	31	35	39	45	65	50	33	F		
9	6	3	3	4	2	1	5	1	1	M	Kaposi's sarcoma	C46
-	1	2	2	-	1	1	1	1	-	F		
1	5	3	2	4	5	1	3	1	1	M	Malignant neoplasm of peripheral nerves and autonomic nervous system	C47
1	3	3	1	3	3	5	4	2	5	F		
5	9	6	11	10	9	16	11	10	3	M	Malignant neoplasm of retroperitoneum and peritoneum	C48
9	7	17	17	28	28	31	19	11	9	F		

Series MB1 no. 32 Table 1

Table 1 Series MB1 no. 32

Table 1 Registrations - *continued*

ICD (10th Revision) number	Site description		All ages	Under 1	1-4	5-9	10-14	15-19	20-24	25-29	30-34	35-39
C49	Malignant neoplasm of other connective and soft tissue	M F	536 469	2 3	4 8	5 8	7 5	19 6	10 9	10 17	17 13	23 16
C50	Malignant neoplasm of breast	M F	245 34,347	- -	- -	- -	- 1	- -	- 19	1 116	1 510	5 1,239
C51	Malignant neoplasm of vulva	F	866	-	-	-	-	-	2	3	12	18
C52	Malignant neoplasm of vagina	F	166	3	-	-	-	-	-	1	2	1
C53	Malignant neoplasm of cervix uteri	F	2,418	-	-	-	-	2	38	151	273	299
C54	Malignant neoplasm of corpus uteri	F	4,678	-	-	-	-	1	2	3	10	37
C55	Malignant neoplasm of uterus, part unspecified	F	276	-	-	-	-	-	-	1	-	7
C56-C57	Malignant neoplasm of ovary and other unspecified female genital organs	F	5,735	-	-	3	8	16	30	57	96	123
C56	Malignant neoplasm of ovary	F	5,635	-	-	3	7	16	30	56	95	120
C57	Malignant neoplasm of other and unspecified female genital organs	F	100	-	-	-	1	-	-	1	1	3
C58	Malignant neoplasm of placenta	F	6	-	-	-	-	-	1	1	3	1
C60	Malignant neoplasm of penis	M	332	-	-	-	-	-	1	1	2	11
C61	Malignant neoplasm of prostate	M	26,027	-	-	1	-	1	1	1	2	9
C62	Malignant neoplasm of testis	M	1,653	1	2	1	4	51	148	239	307	317
C63	Malignant neoplasm of other and unspecified male genital organs	M	54	-	-	1	-	-	-	-	-	2
C64	Malignant neoplasm of kidney, except renal pelvis	M F	2,701 1,648	5 6	20 24	6 7	- -	1 2	4 2	7 6	19 13	31 22
C65	Malignant neoplasm of renal pelvis	M F	203 121	- -	- -	- -	- -	- -	- -	- -	- -	2 1
C66	Malignant neoplasm of ureter	M F	166 92	- -	- -	- -	- -	- -	- -	- -	- -	1 1
C67	Malignant neoplasm of bladder	M F	6,317 2,515	- -	2 -	- -	1 -	2 1	2 -	7 8	11 7	19 9
C68	Malignant neoplasm of other and unspecified urinery organs	M F	83 28	- -	- -	- -	- -	- -	- -	1 1	- -	- -
C69	Malignant neoplasm of eye and adnexa	M F	186 158	3 4	10 11	1 -	1 1	1 2	1 -	3 -	4 1	6 5
C70	Malignant neoplasm of meninges	M F	25 49	- -	1 -	- -	1 -	1 -	- -	1 -	1 1	2 1
C71	Malignant neoplasm of brain	M F	2,032 1,505	9 5	41 32	48 41	47 33	23 24	26 17	55 37	75 41	86 50
C72	Malignant neoplasm of spinal cord, cranial nerves and other parts of central nervous system	M F	55 52	2 -	7 5	5 2	4 7	2 2	2 3	3 1	2 -	1 4
C73	Malignant neoplasm of thyroid gland	M F	316 862	- -	- -	1 2	3 10	4 8	10 21	13 72	18 68	21 91
C74	Malignant neoplasm of adrenal gland	M F	79 98	7 9	9 9	5 3	1 2	2 2	- -	- 1	2 2	1 4
C75	Malignant neoplasm of other endocrine glands and related structures	M F	39 34	1 -	1 2	1 2	3 1	1 -	4 1	2 2	1 -	3 2

40-44	45-49	50-54	55-59	60-64	65-69	70-74	75-79	80-84	85 and over	Sex	Site description	ICD (10th Revision) number
21	23	43	38	49	60	62	55	47	41	M	Malignant neoplasm of other connective and soft tissue	C49
25	30	34	36	32	35	44	54	48	46	F		
2	9	15	26	26	30	52	25	30	23	M	Malignant neoplasm of breast	C50
1,991	2,778	4,678	4,222	3,847	3,037	3,249	3,284	2,475	2,901	F		
34	42	52	38	58	78	119	121	123	166	F	Malignant neoplasm of vulva	C51
5	4	17	10	17	15	14	30	20	27	F	Malignant neoplasm of vagina	C52
286	228	183	151	137	144	154	177	113	82	F	Malignant neoplasm of cervix uteri	C53
83	160	423	640	738	680	603	544	401	353	F	Malignant neoplasm of corpus uteri	C54
8	11	19	25	30	23	25	40	28	59	F	Malignant neoplasm of uterus, part unspecified	C55
175	340	540	629	667	688	709	701	520	433	F	Malignant neoplasm of ovary and other unspecified female genital organs	C56-C57
174	339	527	615	655	674	701	686	512	425	F	Malignant neoplasm of ovary	C56
1	1	13	14	12	14	8	15	8	8	F	Malignant neoplasm of other and unspecified female genital organs	C57
-	-	-	-	-	-	-	-	-	-	F	Malignant neoplasm of placenta	C58
20	20	22	35	43	29	49	49	27	23	M	Malignant neoplasm of penis	C60
18	110	557	1,438	2,808	4,587	5,319	5,177	3,372	2,626	M	Malignant neoplasm of prostate	C61
213	138	94	55	27	16	16	12	7	5	M	Malignant neoplasm of testis	C62
-	4	2	3	6	8	11	8	3	6	M	Malignant neoplasm of other and unspecified male genital organs	C63
80	121	241	267	320	412	396	375	228	168	M	Malignant neoplasm of kidney, except renal pelvis	C64
35	60	125	138	164	225	207	246	182	184	F		
7	6	8	15	29	42	38	32	12	12	M	Malignant neoplasm of renal pelvis	C65
1	5	1	11	14	13	21	19	19	16	F		
-	1	5	10	22	24	34	38	25	6	M	Malignant neoplasm of ureter	C66
1	1	3	3	7	11	24	23	5	13	F		
49	85	220	388	617	856	1,120	1,261	881	796	M	Malignant neoplasm of bladder	C67
21	36	69	111	172	246	365	471	444	555	F		
-	1	2	5	9	13	13	16	15	8	M	Malignant neoplasm of other and unspecified urinery organs	C68
1	-	2	2	2	2	4	3	-	11	F		
6	10	19	17	26	21	21	19	11	6	M	Malignant neoplasm of eye and adnexa	C69
2	7	12	17	13	23	14	22	12	12	F		
-	1	1	2	1	5	4	1	1	2	M	Malignant neoplasm of meninges	C70
3	3	1	4	4	5	5	6	8	8	F		
86	119	187	199	215	255	228	194	99	40	M	Malignant neoplasm of brain	C71
71	77	97	125	149	175	192	153	101	85	F		
2	4	3	3	3	3	2	4	2	1	M	Malignant neoplasm of spinal cord, cranial nerves and other parts of central nervous system	C72
2	1	5	3	5	1	4	1	5	1	F		
23	25	22	32	25	33	25	27	23	11	M	Malignant neoplasm of thyroid gland	C73
72	63	92	65	61	44	62	45	38	48	F		
2	5	8	2	6	6	4	12	6	1	M	Malignant neoplasm of adrenal gland	C74
4	8	5	10	9	10	4	12	3	1	F		
1	2	1	2	4	3	5	3	-	1	M	Malignant neoplasm of other endocrine glands and related structures	C75
4	-	3	1	6	1	6	1	1	1	F		

Table 1 Series MB1 no. 32

Table 1 Registrations - *continued*

ICD (10th Revision) number	Site description		All ages	Age group								
				Under 1	1-4	5-9	10-14	15-19	20-24	25-29	30-34	35-39
C76	Malignant neoplasm of other and ill-defined sites	M F	**207** **327**	2 1	2 1	1 2	2 4	3 -	2 1	3 2	10 3	6 8
C77	Secondary and unspecified malignant neoplasm of lymph nodes	M F	**363** **285**	- -	- -	1 1	- -	- 1	- 1	1 2	5 1	9 7
C78	Secondary malignant neoplasm of respiratory and digestive organs	M F	**1,901** **2,186**	- -	- -	- -	- -	1 -	- 1	1 4	5 11	12 16
C79	Secondary malignant neoplasm of other sites	M F	**891** **884**	- -	1 -	- 1	2 -	1 1	- -	1 4	4 4	6 5
C80	Malignant neoplasm without specification of site	M F	**2,300** **3,040**	- -	- 1	- -	- -	1 1	4 2	4 4	11 8	12 16
C81	Hodgkin's disease	M F	**669** **507**	- -	2 2	10 4	14 20	41 39	77 51	66 61	66 56	72 43
C82-C85	Non-Hodgkin's lymphoma	M F	**4,146** **3,648**	2 -	9 5	17 4	17 10	35 23	30 25	41 43	96 60	113 80
C82	Follicular (nodular) non-Hodgkin's lymphoma	M F	**524** **558**	- -	- -	- -	1 -	1 -	- 2	5 4	17 13	18 12
C83	Diffuse non-Hodgkin's lymphoma lymphoma	M F	**1,487** **1,196**	2 -	6 4	8 4	8 2	15 18	14 10	20 12	31 13	44 29
C84	Peripheral and cutaneous T-cell lymphomas	M F	**273** **176**	- -	1 -	- -	- 1	6 -	2 1	3 6	10 10	9 9
C85	Other and unspecified types on non-Hodgkin's lymphoma	M F	**1,862** **1,718**	- -	2 1	9 -	8 7	13 5	14 12	13 21	38 24	42 30
C88	Malignant immunoproliferative diseases	M F	**133** **74**	- -	1 -	- -	- -	- -	- -	- -	- -	- -
C90	Multiple myeloma and malignant plasma cell neoplasms	M F	**1,528** **1,331**	- -	- -	- -	- -	- -	- -	- 1	3 1	7 10
C91-C95	All leukaemias	M F	**3,159** **2,439**	11 13	83 76	50 49	44 39	41 21	44 23	42 36	50 33	77 37
C91	Lymphoid leukaemia	M F	**1,632** **1,163**	4 8	71 64	41 40	34 24	22 7	11 12	11 10	14 6	24 9
C92	Myeloid leukaemia	M F	**1,368** **1,137**	7 4	11 10	8 9	10 15	15 13	28 11	27 24	35 26	52 25
C93	Monocytic leukaemia	M F	**42** **39**	- 1	1 -	1 -	- -	2 -	1 -	1 2	1 1	1 1
C94	Other leukaemias of specified cell type	M F	**21** **11**	- -	- -	- -	- -	- -	2 -	1 -	- -	- -
C95	Leukaemia of unspecified cell type	M F	**96** **89**	- -	- 2	- -	- -	2 1	2 -	2 -	- -	- 2
C96	Other and unspecified malignant neoplasms of lymphoid, haematopoietic and related tissue	M F	**19** **15**	- -	3 1	1 1	- -	- -	- -	- -	- 1	3 -
C97	Malignant neoplasms of independent (primary) multiple sites	M F	**-** **-**	- -	- -	- -	- -	- -	- -	- -	- -	- -
D00	Carcinoma in situ of oral cavity, oesophagus and stomach	M F	**109** **88**	- -	- -	- -	- -	- 1	- 1	- -	- -	- -
D01	Carcinoma in situ of other and unspecified digestive organs	M F	**195** **180**	- -	- -	- -	- -	1 -	- -	3 2	2 2	3 6
D02	Carcinoma in situ of middle ear and respiratory system	M F	**163** **49**	- -	- -	- -	- -	- -	- -	- -	1 -	- -
D03	Melanoma in situ	M F	**760** **1,112**	- -	- -	- -	- 2	4 5	4 16	16 27	17 39	25 56

40-44	45-49	50-54	55-59	60-64	65-69	70-74	75-79	80-84	85 and over		Site description	ICD (10th Revision) number
4	6	8	15	13	15	28	23	32	32	M	Malignant neoplasm of other and	C76
8	11	19	11	10	26	40	43	45	92	F	ill-defined sites	
17	23	28	29	48	56	48	49	29	20	M	Secondary and unspecified malignant	C77
14	7	16	32	31	32	40	34	28	38	F	neoplasm of lymph nodes	
29	28	79	116	194	221	337	383	279	216	M	Secondary malignant neoplasm of	C78
22	47	75	108	152	209	334	403	372	432	F	respiratory and digestive organs	
13	18	44	62	85	114	153	157	138	92	M	Secondary malignant neoplasm of	C79
7	29	38	58	71	113	145	163	119	126	F	other sites	
24	35	89	121	174	270	371	469	372	343	M	Malignant neoplasm without	C80
32	42	74	131	181	276	412	501	533	826	F	specification of site	
50	42	45	43	37	30	30	23	13	8	M	Hodgkin's disease	C81
34	19	13	24	34	35	27	19	14	12	F		
158	207	342	407	454	542	551	512	349	264	M	Non-Hodgkin's lymphoma	C82-C85
120	136	252	301	356	393	467	544	434	395	F		
32	49	69	74	70	59	49	43	24	13	M	Follicular (nodular) non-Hodgkin's	C82
32	40	68	74	79	63	51	63	41	16	F	lymphoma	
52	62	135	142	154	205	224	174	112	79	M	Diffuse non-Hodgkin's	C83
37	39	70	94	113	123	181	196	134	117	F	lymphoma	
15	11	26	31	27	35	26	29	24	18	M	Peripheral and cutaneous T-cell	C84
9	8	13	18	16	26	15	16	10	18	F	lymphomas	
59	85	112	160	203	243	252	266	189	154	M	Other and unspecified types on non-	C85
42	49	101	115	148	181	220	269	249	244	F	Hodgkin's lymphoma	
-	1	6	9	9	14	23	28	20	22	M	Malignant immunoproliferative	C88
1	1	2	3	4	5	11	17	14	16	F	diseases	
29	39	74	125	172	232	265	251	203	128	M	Multiple myeloma and malignant	C90
17	27	55	87	116	156	180	230	223	228	F	plasma cell neoplasms	
63	94	174	207	293	362	400	477	315	332	M	All leukaemias	C91-C95
45	67	113	145	131	212	296	341	317	445	F		
24	42	79	126	163	205	210	232	149	170	M	Lymphoid leukaemia	C91
12	28	39	61	61	108	137	160	157	220	F		
34	48	86	70	119	142	169	224	142	141	M	Myeloid leukaemia	C92
32	35	69	79	65	96	146	158	134	186	F		
1	2	4	3	3	6	4	5	5	1	M	Monocytic leukaemia	C93
1	2	3	2	1	3	2	8	2	10	F		
2	-	2	2	3	1	5	-	3	-	M	Other leukaemias of specified cell	C94
-	1	1	-	-	1	4	1	1	2	F	type	
2	2	3	6	5	8	12	16	16	20	M	Leukaemia of unspecified cell type	C95
-	1	1	3	4	4	7	14	23	27	F		
-	-	-	1	2	-	3	3	-	3	M	Other and unspecified malignant	C96
-	1	-	1	-	3	1	3	1	2	F	neoplasms of lymphoid, haematopoietic and related tissue	
-	-	-	-	-	-	-	-	-	-	M	Malignant neoplasms of independent	C97
-	-	-	-	-	-	-	-	-	-	F	(primary) multiple sites	
1	4	9	9	18	13	17	24	12	2	M	Carcinoma in situ of oral cavity,	D00
1	2	2	9	3	9	7	22	14	17	F	oesophagus and stomach	
6	7	2	19	19	29	37	28	27	12	M	Carcinoma in situ of other and	D01
4	8	7	19	18	20	22	28	22	22	F	unspecified digestive organs	
2	3	17	17	23	26	25	30	17	2	M	Carcinoma in situ of middle ear and	D02
-	1	6	7	9	4	9	8	2	3	F	respiratory system	
32	32	64	74	80	95	110	98	61	48	M	Melanoma in situ	D03
71	74	106	97	97	120	128	101	97	76	F		

Table 1 Registrations - *continued*

ICD (10th Revision) number	Site description		All ages	Age group Under 1	1-4	5-9	10-14	15-19	20-24	25-29	30-34	35-39
D04	Carcinoma in situ of skin	M F	1,890 3,741	- -	- -	- -	- -	- -	- -	- 3	6 5	16 10
D05	Carcinoma in situ of breast	M F	17 3,019	- -	- -	- -	- -	- -	- -	- 13	- 28	- 79
D06	Carcinoma in situ of cervix uteri	F	19,517	-	-	-	-	218	3,450	5,159	4,592	2,823
D07	Carcinoma in situ of other and unspecified genital organs	M F	406 611	- -	- -	- -	- -	- 3	4 9	4 18	5 45	7 76
D09	Carcinoma in situ of other and unspecified sites	M F	2,243 787	- -	- -	- -	- -	- -	5 2	2 1	9 1	22 4
D33	Benign neoplasm of brain and other parts of central nervous system	M F	235 249	- -	1 3	1 -	4 3	4 8	5 7	8 7	18 10	23 25
D35.2	Benign neoplasm of pituitary gland	M F	201 156	- -	- -	- -	1 1	1 -	3 3	3 6	11 19	9 9
D35.3	Benign neoplasm of craniopharyngeal duct	M F	- -	- -	- -	- -	- -	- -	- -	- -	- -	- -
D35.4	Benign neoplasm of pineal gland	M F	- -	- -	- -	- -	- -	- -	- -	- -	- -	- -
D37	Neoplasm of uncertain or unknown behaviour of oral cavity and digestive organs	M F	654 691	- 1	- -	- -	5 12	6 16	6 11	5 12	5 18	13 14
D38	Neoplasm of uncertain or unknown behaviour of middle ear and respiratory and intrathoracic organs	M F	71 68	- -	- 2	- -	- -	- -	- -	1 -	2 1	3 1
D39	Neoplasm of uncertain or unknown behaviour of female genital organs	F	303	-	1	1	6	9	11	23	21	28
D40	Neoplasm of uncertain or unknown behaviour of male genital organs	M	93	2	2	2	-	2	5	9	4	7
D41	Neoplasm of uncertain or unknown behaviour of urinary organs	M F	1,859 746	1 -	- -	- -	- -	- -	2 -	13 2	10 6	14 7
D42	Neoplasm of uncertain or unknown behaviour of meninges	M F	18 23	- -	- -	- 1	- -	- -	1 1	- -	- -	- 3
D43	Neoplasm of uncertain or unknown behaviour of brain and central nervous system	M F	259 249	2 -	1 1	4 4	5 4	5 4	1 3	11 2	9 2	8 19
D44	Neoplasm of uncertain or unknown behaviour of endocrine glands	M F	90 103	- -	1 1	3 3	1 2	3 6	4 3	1 4	2 6	7 9
D45	Polycythaemia vera	M F	199 156	- -	- -	- -	- -	1 -	- -	1 2	5 1	3 3
D46	Myelodysplastic syndromes	M F	1,104 1,005	- -	1 1	- 1	2 -	- 3	1 3	1 4	2 3	4 1
D47	Other neoplasms of uncertain or unknown behaviour of lymphoid, haematopoietic and related tissue	M F	872 1,009	1 -	- -	1 -	1 2	- 1	2 5	4 8	4 6	12 19
D48	Neoplasm of uncertain or unknown behaviour of other and unspecified sites	M F	243 367	8 2	- 2	2 5	4 4	5 9	11 20	7 14	12 19	16 24
O01	Hydatidiform mole	F	241	-	-	-	-	24	34	62	60	38

Series MB1 no. 32 Table 1

40-44	45-49	50-54	55-59	60-64	65-69	70-74	75-79	80-84	85 and over		Site description	ICD (10th Revision) number
23	34	74	131	174	247	325	361	302	197	M	Carcinoma in situ of skin	D04
23	47	90	148	252	453	572	704	665	769	F		
1	1	1	2	-	1	5	2	2	2	M	Carcinoma in situ of breast	D05
134	258	784	580	509	224	177	127	62	44	F		
1,411	743	470	285	217	82	29	19	13	6	F	Carcinoma in situ of cervix uteri	D06
6	8	20	28	58	101	92	49	17	7	M	Carcinoma in situ of other and unspecified genital organs	D07
69	71	76	53	47	35	35	43	12	19	F		
24	58	88	175	239	335	418	445	272	151	M	Carcinoma in situ of other and unspecified sites	D09
12	16	49	58	73	103	145	133	103	87	F		
25	36	26	26	10	19	14	12	1	2	M	Benign neoplasm of brain and other parts of central nervous system	D33
21	19	27	27	26	20	23	13	4	6	F		
10	21	23	18	19	28	26	15	11	2	M	Benign neoplasm of pituitary gland	D35.2
12	13	13	15	17	20	11	11	4	2	F		
-	-	-	-	-	-	-	-	-	-	M	Benign neoplasm of craniopharyngeal duct	D35.3
-	-	-	-	-	-	-	-	-	-	F		
-	-	-	-	-	-	-	-	-	-	M	Benign neoplasm of pineal gland	D35.4
-	-	-	-	-	-	-	-	-	-	F		
7	16	41	51	75	93	124	104	54	49	M	Neoplasm of uncertain or unknown behaviour of oral cavity and digestive organs	D37
26	24	34	37	60	77	83	97	83	86	F		
-	4	3	4	6	6	12	15	6	9	M	Neoplasm of uncertain or unknown behaviour of middle ear and respiratory and intrathoracic organs	D38
1	3	2	4	4	11	16	9	6	8	F		
24	39	30	22	23	16	20	11	10	8	F	Neoplasm of uncertain or unknown behaviour of female genital organs	D39
6	5	8	8	2	6	10	7	3	5	M	Neoplasm of uncertain or unknown behaviour of male genital organs	D40
34	46	106	154	218	296	307	300	223	135	M	Neoplasm of uncertain or unknown behaviour of urinary organs	D41
12	16	45	54	84	79	151	112	94	84	F		
2	2	4	1	2	1	1	3	1	-	M	Neoplasm of uncertain or unknown behaviour of meninges	D42
1	2	-	2	1	5	4	2	-	1	F		
19	9	13	11	22	16	30	34	32	27	M	Neoplasm of uncertain or unknown behaviour of brain and central nervous system	D43
10	10	4	14	12	12	39	38	38	33	F		
3	8	5	10	8	9	7	8	4	6	M	Neoplasm of uncertain or unknown behaviour of endocrine glands	D44
5	4	4	6	11	6	7	12	5	9	F		
12	6	9	21	28	24	23	39	18	9	M	Polycythaemia vera	D45
5	3	14	12	11	23	19	25	19	19	F		
7	8	17	35	46	97	158	239	219	267	M	Myelodysplastic syndromes	D46
9	7	17	21	32	69	92	168	210	364	F		
18	30	44	69	92	95	130	155	126	88	M	Other neoplasms of uncertain or unknown behaviour of lymphoid, haematopoietic and related tissue	D47
23	29	58	41	64	95	148	187	148	175	F		
15	18	15	19	14	17	19	27	12	22	M	Neoplasm of uncertain or unknown behaviour of other and unspecified sites	D48
25	25	38	34	20	26	14	29	25	32	F		
10	7	6	-	-	-	-	-	-	-	F	Hydatidiform mole	O01

Table 2 Series MB1 no. 32

Table 2 Estimated resident population:
sex and age as at 30 June 2001

(Figures in thousands)

Area		All ages	Under 1	1-4	5-9	10-14	15-19	20-24	25-29	30-34	35-39
England	M	24,143.9	284.6	1,210.5	1,597.1	1,656.4	1,556.1	1,475.7	1,674.0	1,934.2	1,931.2
	F	25,245.8	272.7	1,152.7	1,519.7	1,578.4	1,484.1	1,488.0	1,656.6	1,926.4	1,970.2
Goverment office for the region											
North East	M	1,221.6	13.1	57.6	80.5	85.6	83.0	75.4	72.5	87.1	95.7
	F	1,297.2	12.6	54.7	76.2	81.9	81.6	75.5	75.4	91.7	99.6
North West	M	3,284.5	38.0	164.6	224.7	239.6	222.3	193.2	206.8	246.7	256.5
	F	3,482.7	36.4	156.0	213.3	228.7	216.8	201.1	212.1	255.1	266.0
Yorkshire and The Humber	M	2,416.8	28.0	120.4	164.2	171.6	163.6	151.8	151.3	181.3	187.3
	F	2,553.7	26.9	115.8	156.7	165.1	157.5	153.7	156.1	187.3	192.3
East Midlands	M	2,058.0	23.0	99.6	136.2	143.7	134.5	124.7	127.6	156.1	162.2
	F	2,124.8	21.7	94.1	128.4	136.2	126.3	120.7	127.2	159.0	164.3
West Midlands	M	2,590.9	30.3	132.8	174.9	185.9	174.6	154.4	167.0	200.3	198.2
	F	2,691.9	29.4	125.5	167.8	177.3	165.8	155.0	164.2	198.3	202.3
East of England	M	2,648.5	31.0	133.5	175.6	179.8	163.1	151.2	170.1	202.5	211.0
	F	2,752.8	30.0	126.6	167.9	171.8	155.2	147.7	169.8	203.4	213.5
London	M	3,598.0	49.7	194.1	230.7	222.4	212.9	254.4	384.8	393.7	319.6
	F	3,709.9	47.4	186.9	220.9	213.4	204.6	277.1	361.1	355.4	324.5
South East	M	3,923.1	45.8	196.1	259.6	266.2	249.8	233.6	252.8	296.7	317.7
	F	4,098.3	43.7	186.2	245.3	251.5	234.5	228.9	250.3	301.8	321.9
South West	M	2,402.6	25.7	111.9	150.6	161.6	152.3	137.0	141.2	169.9	183.0
	F	2,534.4	24.6	106.9	143.2	152.5	141.8	128.4	140.4	174.4	185.9

Series MB1 no. 32 Table 2

England, government offices for the regions

40-44	45-49	50-54	55-59	60-64	65-69	70-74	75-79	80-84	85 and over		Area
1,736.0	**1,553.3**	**1,665.9**	**1,401.1**	**1,174.7**	**1,036.8**	**888.2**	**687.2**	**414.1**	**266.9**	**M**	**England**
1,751.3	**1,573.8**	**1,694.1**	**1,427.7**	**1,217.9**	**1,120.9**	**1,061.9**	**954.9**	**703.4**	**691.0**	**F**	
											Goverment office for the region
90.3	83.8	88.1	71.2	63.6	57.8	48.5	36.6	20.2	11.4	M	North East
93.5	84.1	88.5	72.0	67.4	63.4	59.8	52.0	36.0	31.5	F	
234.7	213.8	234.0	193.6	168.3	147.0	122.4	92.6	53.4	32.5	M	North West
240.6	216.8	235.0	196.5	175.2	160.1	151.0	133.2	96.6	92.4	F	
173.2	157.1	170.8	142.1	121.0	106.6	89.6	70.3	41.1	25.6	M	Yorkshire and The Humber
175.8	157.7	172.3	142.9	126.6	117.6	110.3	97.8	71.6	69.7	F	
147.6	134.9	148.9	126.8	102.9	90.4	78.7	61.9	36.3	21.8	M	East Midlands
148.3	135.1	148.2	127.2	104.8	96.3	91.0	81.3	58.9	55.6	F	
180.5	166.5	179.4	157.5	132.1	113.7	98.1	74.2	44.0	26.3	M	West Midlands
181.4	167.2	179.0	158.4	134.7	122.5	115.8	102.9	75.6	68.9	F	
192.8	173.2	190.6	161.1	131.6	118.7	102.6	79.6	48.5	31.8	M	East of England
190.4	175.4	194.6	163.7	135.1	125.7	119.0	106.7	78.6	77.7	F	
259.1	208.9	198.7	157.9	136.8	119.3	99.8	76.0	47.2	32.0	M	London
260.1	215.0	210.5	169.6	145.4	128.9	120.3	108.6	79.0	81.1	F	
290.2	259.5	280.2	236.3	190.0	168.3	145.1	113.2	72.1	49.8	M	South East
289.5	261.3	285.4	239.7	196.2	182.3	173.3	158.6	121.6	126.5		
167.5	155.6	175.1	154.7	128.2	115.0	103.3	82.9	51.4	35.7	M	South West
171.7	161.2	180.6	157.8	132.5	124.1	121.5	113.8	85.5	87.6	F	

Table 3 Series MB1 no. 32

Table 3 Rates per 100,000 population of newly diagnosed cases of cancer: site, sex and age, 2001

ICD (10th Revision) number	Site description	Sex	All ages	Under 1	1-4	5-9	10-14	15-19	20-24	25-29	30-34	35-39
	All registrations	M	625.7	24.6	18.2	11.8	12.8	20.9	35.2	48.0	66.9	93.0
		F	673.9	18.7	17.6	10.5	12.9	35.8	266.6	380.4	343.2	318.4
C00-C97	All cancers	M	577.3	19.7	17.7	11.0	11.4	18.9	31.5	42.7	60.5	83.1
		F	537.3	17.6	16.7	9.5	10.6	15.2	26.1	56.3	89.6	153.3
C00-C97 xC44	All cancers excluding nmsc	M	466.0	19.7	17.7	10.7	11.1	18.1	30.4	38.9	51.9	67.4
		F	444.2	17.2	16.7	9.4	10.3	14.2	24.2	50.7	80.6	133.8
C00-C14	Malignant neoplasm of lip, mouth and pharynx	M	10.8	0.4	-	0.1	0.2	0.4	0.6	1.0	1.1	2.4
		F	5.8	-	-	0.2	0.1	0.4	0.5	0.9	0.9	1.5
C00	Malignant neoplasm of lip	M	0.7	-	-	-	-	-	-	-	0.2	0.2
		F	0.3	-	-	-	-	-	0.1	-	-	-
C01	Malignant neoplasm of base of tongue	M	0.8	-	-	-	-	-	-	-	-	0.1
		F	0.2	-	-	-	-	-	-	-	-	-
C02	Malignant neoplasm of other and unspecified parts of tongue	M	1.8	-	-	-	-	0.1	0.2	0.4	0.5	0.6
		F	1.2	-	-	-	-	-	0.1	0.2	0.4	0.4
C03	Malignant neoplasm of gum	M	0.4	0.4	-	-	-	0.1	-	-	0.1	0.2
		F	0.3	-	-	-	-	0.1	-	-	-	-
C04	Malignant neoplasm of floor of mouth	M	1.0	-	-	-	-	-	-	-	0.1	0.1
		F	0.4	-	-	-	-	-	-	-	0.1	0.1
C05	Malignant neoplasm of palate	M	0.5	-	-	0.1	-	-	-	-	0.1	0.1
		F	0.4	-	-	-	-	-	0.1	0.2	0.2	0.1
C06	Malignant neoplasm of other and unspecified parts of mouth	M	0.8	-	-	-	-	-	0.1	0.1	-	0.2
		F	0.6	-	-	-	-	-	-	0.1	-	-
C07	Malignant neoplasm of parotid gland	M	0.8	-	-	-	0.1	0.1	-	0.2	0.2	0.3
		F	0.6	-	-	0.1	0.1	0.1	0.1	0.3	0.1	0.5
C08	Malignant neoplasm of other and unspecified major salivory glands	M	0.2	-	-	-	0.1	0.1	0.1	0.1	-	0.2
		F	0.2	-	-	0.1	0.1	-	-	-	-	0.2
C09	Malignant neoplasm of tonsil	M	1.4	-	-	-	-	-	-	-	0.1	0.3
		F	0.5	-	-	-	-	-	-	-	-	0.1
C10	Malignant neoplasm of oropharynx	M	0.4	-	-	-	-	-	-	-	-	-
		F	0.1	-	-	-	-	-	-	-	0.1	-
C11	Malignant neoplasm of nasopharynx	M	0.4	-	-	0.1	0.1	0.1	0.2	0.2	0.1	0.2
		F	0.3	-	-	-	-	0.2	0.1	0.1	0.1	0.2
C12	Malignant neoplasm of piriform sinus	M	0.7	-	-	-	-	-	-	0.1	-	-
		F	0.1	-	-	-	-	-	-	-	-	-
C13	Malignant neoplasm of hypopharynx hypopharynx	M	0.3	-	-	-	-	-	-	-	-	-
		F	0.3	-	-	-	-	-	-	-	0.1	-
C14	Malignant neoplasm of other and ill-defined sites in the lip, oral cavity and pharynx	M	0.5	-	-	-	-	-	-	0.1	-	0.1
		F	0.2	-	-	0.1	-	-	-	-	-	0.1
C15	Malignant neoplasm of oesophagus	M	15.8	-	-	-	-	0.1	-	0.1	0.4	0.8
		F	9.0	-	-	-	-	-	-	-	0.3	0.5
C16	Malignant neoplasm of stomach	M	19.6	0.4	-	-	-	0.1	0.1	0.3	1.0	0.9
		F	10.4	-	-	-	-	0.1	-	0.2	0.4	1.1
C17	Malignant neoplasm of small intestine	M	1.3	-	-	-	-	-	-	0.2	0.2	0.3
		F	1.1	-	-	-	-	-	0.1	-	0.1	0.2
C18-C20	Malignant neoplasm of colon and rectum	M	61.4	-	-	0.1	0.1	0.1	1.1	0.7	1.9	5.0
		F	50.3	-	-	-	-	0.3	0.4	0.5	0.9	2.4	3.6
C18	Malignant neoplasm of colon	M	36.7	-	-	0.1	0.1	0.1	0.7	0.5	1.3	2.9
		F	34.4	-	-	-	-	0.3	0.3	0.3	0.7	1.4	2.2
C19	Malignant neoplasm of rectosigmoid junction	M	5.0	-	-	-	-	-	0.1	0.1	0.1	0.2
		F	3.4	-	-	-	-	-	-	0.1	-	0.4

England
Registered by May 2004

40-44	45-49	50-54	55-59	60-64	65-69	70-74	75-79	80-84	85 and over	Sex	Site description	ICD (10th Revision) number
146.9	245.6	449.8	802.6	1,342.5	2,071.2	2,856.5	3,803.1	4,344.3	5,170.1	M	All registrations	
365.6	489.7	731.6	912.3	1,169.5	1,359.7	1,772.8	2,175.5	2,480.0	2,861.2	F		
132.4	222.6	414.4	739.6	1,244.3	1,921.3	2,643.7	3,512.8	4,001.4	4,779.6	M	All cancers	C00-C97
256.6	399.4	620.5	804.0	1,038.9	1,225.1	1,607.9	1,976.7	2,247.4	2,590.5	F		
101.2	174.5	326.9	596.1	1,018.2	1,571.7	2,174.9	2,835.3	3,154.5	3,679.8	M	All cancers excluding nmsc	C00-C97 xC44
223.3	345.5	539.1	691.3	880.3	1,014.3	1,322.7	1,603.4	1,774.3	1,984.6	F		
6.2	12.4	20.7	28.8	30.3	30.3	30.4	38.7	36.9	34.1	M	Malignant neoplasm of lip, mouth	C00-C14
4.4	5.8	8.3	10.3	13.3	12.0	16.7	17.3	16.3	24.9	F	and pharynx	
0.3	0.6	0.7	0.8	1.4	1.4	2.8	4.2	3.9	4.9	M	Malignant neoplasm of lip	C00
0.1	0.2	0.1	0.3	0.6	0.9	0.8	1.2	1.4	3.0	F		
0.3	1.3	2.0	2.5	2.6	1.9	1.7	1.5	1.9	1.9	M	Malignant neoplasm of base of	C01
0.2	0.6	0.5	0.9	0.4	0.4	0.7	0.8	0.6	0.1	F	tongue	
1.1	2.0	3.5	4.1	5.2	5.8	5.5	6.3	5.3	4.1	M	Malignant neoplasm of other and	C02
0.9	1.0	2.1	2.0	2.8	2.7	2.7	3.7	2.6	5.6	F	unspecified parts of tongue	
0.5	0.6	0.5	1.0	1.0	0.8	0.8	2.2	2.2	3.0	M	Malignant neoplasm of gum	C03
0.1	0.2	0.1	0.6	0.9	1.0	1.3	1.7	0.9	1.9	F		
0.7	1.0	2.5	3.6	3.2	3.7	1.9	2.5	1.4	0.7	M	Malignant neoplasm of floor of	C04
0.2	0.6	0.9	0.6	1.1	0.9	1.1	1.4	1.4	1.4	F	mouth	
0.2	0.4	1.0	2.0	1.4	1.2	1.1	1.3	1.7	2.2	M	Malignant neoplasm of palate	C05
0.5	0.6	0.5	0.6	0.7	0.3	1.6	1.5	1.0	1.0	F		
0.2	0.6	1.2	2.1	2.9	2.3	2.4	3.2	3.6	5.2	M	Malignant neoplasm of other and	C06
0.3	0.4	0.5	0.7	1.4	1.2	1.7	1.9	2.6	4.5	F	unspecified parts of mouth	
0.5	0.7	1.0	1.1	1.1	1.5	2.7	5.4	7.2	4.9	M	Malignant neoplasm of parotid gland	C07
0.6	0.3	0.6	0.6	1.5	1.0	1.9	1.5	1.1	2.7	F		
0.1	-	0.3	0.4	0.4	1.2	0.5	1.0	0.7	0.7	M	Malignant neoplasm of other and	C08
0.2	0.2	0.2	0.5	0.2	0.4	0.7	0.6	0.6	0.9	F	unspecified major salivory glands	
1.5	3.2	3.5	4.5	3.5	2.7	3.3	3.1	1.2	1.5	M	Malignant neoplasm of tonsil	C09
0.6	0.5	1.1	1.3	1.5	1.2	0.9	0.8	1.1	0.6	F		
0.1	0.3	1.0	1.6	1.2	1.4	1.5	1.2	1.7	0.7	M	Malignant neoplasm of oropharynx	C10
0.1	0.2	0.2	0.1	0.3	0.3	0.3	0.3	0.3	0.3	F		
0.3	0.6	1.1	1.0	1.2	1.0	1.0	0.9	1.4	0.4	M	Malignant neoplasm of nasopharynx	C11
0.4	0.4	0.5	0.6	0.6	0.1	0.2	0.4	0.3	0.6	F		
-	0.3	1.3	2.0	2.6	2.9	2.6	2.6	1.4	0.7	M	Malignant neoplasm of piriform	C12
0.1	0.3	0.3	0.5	0.4	0.3	0.5	0.1	0.3	0.3	F	sinus	
0.2	0.3	0.5	0.7	0.9	1.0	1.5	1.2	1.2	1.9	M	Malignant neoplasm of hypopharynx	C13
0.1	0.2	0.2	0.6	0.6	0.6	1.6	0.5	1.4	0.7	F	hypopharynx	
0.1	0.5	0.6	1.4	1.5	1.6	1.2	2.3	1.9	1.1	M	Malignant neoplasm of other and	C14
-	0.1	0.4	0.4	0.4	0.8	0.7	0.9	0.9	1.2	F	ill-defined sites in the lip, oral cavity and pharynx	
2.7	7.3	14.9	25.7	40.0	49.4	73.9	91.5	110.4	106.8	M	Malignant neoplasm of oesophagus	C15
0.6	2.9	5.3	7.5	14.2	17.6	29.1	44.0	53.3	77.0	F		
3.5	6.1	11.3	21.1	38.0	59.4	101.0	130.5	164.0	194.9	M	Malignant neoplasm of stomach	C16
2.2	3.3	4.7	6.7	14.0	23.5	37.8	49.1	68.2	78.9	F		
0.5	0.7	1.4	2.4	3.2	4.7	5.3	7.3	5.3	8.6	M	Malignant neoplasm of small	C17
0.6	0.4	0.6	1.7	2.7	2.9	3.3	4.3	5.0	5.5	F	intestine	
10.5	19.2	44.4	82.7	134.8	212.6	298.1	390.7	449.4	491.3	M	Malignant neoplasm of colon	C18-C20
9.3	18.4	31.9	55.5	85.7	124.7	176.9	236.5	272.5	327.1	F	and rectum	
5.4	9.6	24.1	41.0	76.0	122.9	179.6	248.4	292.7	319.3	M	Malignant neoplasm of colon	C18
5.8	13.1	19.4	35.7	56.3	83.9	122.2	164.1	189.5	233.1	F		
0.7	2.3	3.1	8.1	12.5	18.5	26.0	30.7	30.2	30.0	M	Malignant neoplasm of rectosigmoid	C19
0.7	1.2	2.6	4.4	6.7	10.1	11.5	16.4	15.8	16.6	F	junction	

Table 3   Rates per 100,000 population - *continued*

ICD (10th Revision) number	Site description		All ages	Age group								
				Under 1	1-4	5-9	10-14	15-19	20-24	25-29	30-34	35-39
C20	Malignant neoplasm of rectum	M	19.8	-	-	-	-	0.1	0.3	0.1	0.5	1.9
		F	12.6	-	-	-	-	0.1	0.2	0.2	1.0	1.0
C21	Malignant neoplasm of anus and anal canal	M	1.1	-	-	-	-	-	-	-	0.2	0.1
		F	1.5	-	-	-	-	-	0.1	0.1	0.2	0.4
C22	Malignant neoplasm of liver and intrahepatic bile ducts	M	5.1	2.1	0.5	-	0.1	0.1	0.1	0.5	0.5	0.5
		F	3.5	1.1	0.3	-	-	0.2	-	0.2	0.1	0.4
C23	Malignant neoplasm of gallbladder	M	0.5	-	-	-	-	-	-	-	-	0.1
		F	1.1	-	-	-	-	-	-	-	-	0.1
C24	Malignant neoplasm of other and unspecified parts of biliary tract	M	1.2	-	-	-	-	-	-	-	0.1	-
		F	1.2	-	0.1	-	-	-	0.1	-	0.1	0.1
C25	Malignant neoplasm of pancreas	M	11.6	-	-	-	-	-	-	0.1	0.3	1.4
		F	11.8	-	-	-	-	0.1	0.1	-	0.2	0.5
C26	Malignant neoplasm of other and ill-defined digestive organs	M	1.0	-	-	-	-	-	-	0.1	-	0.2
		F	1.3	-	-	0.1	-	-	-	-	0.1	0.1
C30	Malignant neoplasm of nasal cavity and middle ear	M	0.4	-	-	0.1	-	-	0.2	-	0.1	0.2
		F	0.3	-	-	-	-	0.1	-	-	0.2	0.2
C31	Malignant neoplasm of accessory sinuses	M	0.4	-	0.1	-	-	0.1	-	-	0.2	0.1
		F	0.2	-	0.1	-	-	-	0.1	0.1	0.1	0.1
C32	Malignant neoplasm of larynx	M	6.1	-	-	-	-	-	-	0.2	0.2	0.5
		F	1.3	-	-	-	-	-	0.1	-	0.1	0.1
C33-C34	Malignant neoplasm of trachea, bronchus and lung	M	76.9	0.4	-	-	-	0.2	0.1	0.5	1.1	2.5
		F	47.4	-	0.1	-	0.1	0.1	0.1	0.4	1.1	2.0
C33	Malignant neoplasm of trachea	M	0.1	-	-	-	-	-	-	-	-	-
		F	0.1	-	-	-	-	-	-	-	-	0.1
C34	Malignant neoplasm of bronchus and lung	M	76.8	0.4	-	-	-	0.2	0.1	0.5	1.1	2.5
		F	47.3	-	0.1	-	0.1	0.1	0.1	0.4	1.1	2.0
C37	Malignant neoplasm of thymus	M	0.1	-	-	-	-	-	-	-	0.1	0.2
		F	0.1	-	-	-	-	-	-	0.1	-	-
C38	Malignant neoplasm of heart, mediastinum and pleura	M	0.6	0.7	0.2	-	0.1	0.1	-	0.3	0.2	0.1
		F	0.4	-	0.1	-	-	-	-	-	0.1	0.1
C39	Malignant neoplasm of other and ill-defined sites in the respiratory system and intrathoracic organs	M	0.0	-	-	-	-	-	-	-	-	-
		F	0.0	-	-	-	-	-	-	-	-	-
C40	Malignant neoplasm of bone and articular cartilage of limbs	M	0.5	-	0.1	0.4	1.1	1.1	0.3	0.4	0.3	0.2
		F	0.4	-	-	0.3	0.5	1.0	0.3	0.2	0.3	0.2
C41	Malignant neoplasm of bone and articular cartilage of other and unspecified sites	M	0.5	-	0.1	0.1	0.2	0.4	0.5	0.3	0.4	0.2
		F	0.5	-	0.2	0.2	0.3	0.3	0.3	0.2	0.3	0.4
C43	Malignant melanoma of skin	M	10.9	-	-	-	0.1	0.6	2.5	3.8	6.2	6.8
		F	13.6	-	-	-	0.1	1.3	5.3	8.8	9.6	12.5
C44	Other malignant neoplasms of skin	M	111.3	-	-	0.3	0.3	0.8	1.1	3.8	8.6	15.7
		F	93.2	0.4	-	0.1	0.3	0.9	1.9	5.6	9.1	19.5
C45	Mesothelioma	M	5.9	-	-	-	-	-	-	0.1	-	0.1
		F	1.3	-	-	-	-	-	-	-	0.1	0.1
C46	Kaposi's sarcoma	M	0.3	-	-	-	-	-	0.1	0.1	0.7	0.5
		F	0.1	-	-	0.1	-	-	-	-	0.2	0.2
C47	Malignant neoplasm of peripheral nerves and autonomic nervous system	M	0.2	-	0.4	0.1	-	0.1	0.1	0.3	0.1	0.2
		F										
C48	Malignant neoplasm of retroperitoneum and peritoneum	M	0.4	-	0.1	0.1	-	0.1	-	0.1	0.1	0.1
		F	0.7	-	-	-	-	-	-	-	0.1	0.3

40-44	45-49	50-54	55-59	60-64	65-69	70-74	75-79	80-84	85 and over		Site description	ICD (10th Revision) number
4.4	7.3	17.1	33.5	46.3	71.2	92.5	111.6	126.5	142.0	M	Malignant neoplasm of rectum	C20
2.8	4.1	9.9	15.5	22.7	30.8	43.1	55.9	67.2	77.3	F		
0.7	0.7	1.6	2.6	2.3	3.2	3.9	4.4	5.3	6.7	M	Malignant neoplasm of anus and anal	C21
0.9	1.7	2.0	1.8	3.3	2.9	5.1	5.2	6.7	6.5	F	canal	
1.4	2.8	4.9	7.7	12.3	15.5	21.8	30.9	29.2	41.2	M	Malignant neoplasm of liver and	C22
0.7	0.5	1.8	3.2	5.4	8.3	12.7	18.9	21.8	19.8	F	intrahepatic bile ducts	
0.1	0.1	0.4	0.7	1.2	2.2	1.4	3.8	3.4	4.9	M	Malignant neoplasm of gallbladder	C23
0.3	0.3	0.7	2.0	1.0	3.5	4.3	5.1	4.8	7.8	F		
0.2	0.3	0.5	2.1	2.6	3.5	5.2	8.1	9.2	13.1	M	Malignant neoplasm of other and	C24
0.4	0.1	0.6	1.2	2.5	1.9	4.4	5.1	7.7	9.3	F	unspecified parts of biliary tract	
2.1	5.5	8.0	14.9	26.9	41.1	51.5	69.0	79.2	115.4	M	Malignant neoplasm of pancreas	C25
2.1	2.5	6.0	11.0	18.8	26.5	41.3	54.7	77.3	87.7	F		
0.2	0.2	0.7	1.0	1.1	2.4	5.6	3.8	9.2	15.4	M	Malignant neoplasm of other and	C26
0.2	0.5	0.5	0.8	1.1	2.6	2.6	4.1	8.0	18.4	F	ill-defined digestive organs	
0.2	0.3	0.6	0.8	0.7	1.3	1.6	1.5	1.2	3.7	M	Malignant neoplasm of nasal cavity	C30
0.2	0.3	0.4	0.6	0.2	1.2	1.2	1.6	1.0	1.2	F	and middle ear	
0.1	0.4	0.5	0.9	0.6	1.0	1.4	1.9	2.2	1.5	M	Malignant neoplasm of accessory	C31
0.1	0.3	0.4	0.3	0.2	0.2	0.5	0.7	1.1	1.2	F	sinuses	
1.2	3.5	8.9	15.1	18.3	24.0	25.6	24.7	24.4	24.7	M	Malignant neoplasm of larynx	C32
0.3	1.0	1.8	2.5	3.4	4.3	4.6	4.0	3.7	4.9	F		
7.0	21.8	45.9	95.9	172.9	269.0	403.7	536.7	560.0	566.6	M	Malignant neoplasm of trachea,	C33-C34
6.1	17.3	35.9	58.7	95.0	131.7	212.0	246.9	233.7	170.8	F	bronchus and lung	
-	0.1	0.1	-	0.3	0.2	0.8	1.3	1.2	0.7	M	Malignant neoplasm of trachea	C33
-	0.1	0.1	0.2	0.2	-	0.6	0.4	0.1	0.3	F		
7.0	21.7	45.7	95.9	172.6	268.8	402.9	535.4	558.8	565.8	M	Malignant neoplasm of bronchus	C34
6.1	17.3	35.8	58.5	94.8	131.7	211.4	246.5	233.6	170.5	F	and lung	
0.1	0.1	0.3	0.1	0.4	0.5	0.2	0.3	-	1.1	M	Malignant neoplasm of thymus	C37
0.2	0.1	0.5	0.1	0.1	0.4	0.4	0.2	0.3	-	F		
0.2	0.2	0.5	0.7	1.0	1.1	2.9	1.9	4.6	4.9	M	Malignant neoplasm of heart,	C38
0.1	0.2	0.4	0.6	0.6	0.6	1.5	2.0	1.8	1.4	F	mediastinum and pleura	
-	-	-	-	-	0.2	0.1	-	-	0.4	M	Malignant neoplasm of other and	C39
-	-	0.1	0.1	-	-	0.1	-	-	-	F	ill-defined sites in the respiratory system and intrathoracic organs	
0.3	0.5	0.3	0.4	0.3	0.3	0.1	1.2	1.2	1.1	M	Malignant neoplasm of bone and	C40
0.1	0.1	0.5	0.4	0.4	0.2	0.4	0.6	0.4	1.4	F	articular cartilage of limbs	
0.3	0.2	0.2	0.8	0.9	0.9	0.8	1.5	2.2	1.9	M	Malignant neoplasm of bone and	C41
0.3	-	0.5	0.5	0.5	0.8	1.1	1.2	1.3	2.2	F	articular cartilage of other and unspecified sites	
9.7	13.6	15.7	18.5	24.2	27.6	29.3	34.5	42.5	49.8	M	Malignant melanoma of skin	C43
15.1	18.7	19.8	22.1	19.7	25.4	26.6	28.6	35.3	30.0	F		
31.2	48.1	87.6	143.5	226.2	349.5	468.8	677.4	846.9	1,099.8	M	Other malignant neoplasms of skin	C44
33.3	53.9	81.5	112.8	158.6	210.7	285.2	373.2	473.1	606.0	F		
0.2	1.5	4.1	9.9	17.9	23.6	27.5	40.6	32.6	27.7	M	Mesothelioma	C45
0.1	0.7	0.8	2.2	2.9	3.5	4.2	6.8	7.1	4.8	F		
0.5	0.4	0.2	0.2	0.3	0.2	0.1	0.7	0.2	0.4	M	Kaposi's sarcoma	C46
-	0.1	0.1	0.1	-	0.1	0.1	0.1	0.1	-	F		
0.1	0.2	0.2	0.1	0.2	0.3	0.5	0.4	0.3	0.7	M	Malignant neoplasm of peripheral	C47
										F	nerves and autonomic nervous system	
0.3	0.6	0.4	0.8	0.9	0.9	1.8	1.6	2.4	1.1	M	Malignant neoplasm of	C48
0.5	0.4	1.0	1.2	2.3	2.5	2.9	2.0	1.6	1.3	F	retroperitoneum and peritoneum	

Table 3 Rates per 100,000 population - *continued*

ICD (10th Revision) number	Site description		All ages	Under 1	1-4	5-9	10-14	15-19	20-24	25-29	30-34	35-39
C49	Malignant neoplasm of other connective and soft tissue	M F	2.2 1.9	0.7 1.1	0.3 0.7	0.3 0.5	0.4 0.3	1.2 0.4	0.7 0.6	0.6 1.0	0.9 0.7	1.2 0.8
C50	Malignant neoplasm of breast	M F	1.0 136.1	- -	- -	- -	- 0.1	- -	- 1.3	0.1 7.0	0.1 26.5	0.3 62.9
C51	Malignant neoplasm of vulva	F	3.4	-	-	-	-	-	0.1	0.2	0.6	0.9
C52	Malignant neoplasm of vagina	F	0.7	1.1	-	-	-	-	-	0.1	0.1	0.1
C53	Malignant neoplasm of cervix uteri	F	9.6	-	-	-	-	0.1	2.6	9.1	14.2	15.2
C54	Malignant neoplasm of corpus uteri	F	18.5	-	-	-	-	0.1	0.1	0.2	0.5	1.9
C55	Malignant neoplasm of uterus, part unspecified	F	1.1	-	-	-	-	-	-	0.1	-	0.4
C56-C57	Malignant neoplasm of ovary and other unspecified female genital organs	F	22.7	-	-	0.2	0.5	1.1	2.0	3.4	5.0	6.2
C56	Malignant neoplasm of ovary	F	22.3	-	-	0.2	0.4	1.1	2.0	3.4	4.9	6.1
C57	Malignant neoplasm of other and unspecified female genital organs	F	0.4	-	-	-	0.1	-	-	0.1	0.1	0.2
C58	Malignant neoplasm of placenta	F	0.0	-	-	-	-	-	0.1	0.1	0.2	0.1
C60	Malignant neoplasm of penis	M	1.4	-	-	-	-	-	0.1	0.1	0.1	0.6
C61	Malignant neoplasm of prostate	M	107.8	-	-	0.1	-	0.1	0.1	0.1	0.1	0.5
C62	Malignant neoplasm of testis	M	6.8	0.4	0.2	0.1	0.2	3.3	10.0	14.3	15.9	16.4
C63	Malignant neoplasm of other and unspecified male genital organs	M	0.2	-	-	0.1	-	-	-	-	-	0.1
C64	Malignant neoplasm of kidney, except renal pelvis	M F	11.2 6.5	1.8 2.2	1.7 2.1	0.4 0.5	- -	0.1 0.1	0.3 0.1	0.4 0.4	1.0 0.7	1.6 1.1
C65	Malignant neoplasm of renal pelvis	M F	0.8 0.5	- -	- -	- -	- -	- -	- -	- -	- -	0.1 0.1
C66	Malignant neoplasm of ureter	M F	0.7 0.4	- -	- -	- -	- -	- -	- -	- -	- -	0.1 0.1
C67	Malignant neoplasm of bladder	M F	26.2 10.0	- -	0.2 -	- -	0.1 -	0.1 0.1	0.1 -	0.4 0.5	0.6 0.4	1.0 0.5
C68	Malignant neoplasm of other and unspecified urinery organs	M F	0.3 0.1	- -	- -	- -	- -	- -	- -	0.1 0.1	- -	- -
C69	Malignant neoplasm of eye and adnexa	M F	0.8 0.6	1.1 1.5	0.8 1.0	0.1 -	0.1 0.1	0.1 0.1	0.1 -	0.2 -	0.2 0.1	0.3 0.3
C70	Malignant neoplasm of meninges	M F	0.1 0.2	- -	0.1 -	- -	0.1 -	0.1 -	- -	0.1 -	0.1 0.1	0.1 0.1
C71	Malignant neoplasm of brain	M F	8.4 6.0	3.2 1.8	3.4 2.8	3.0 2.7	2.8 2.1	1.5 1.6	1.8 1.1	3.3 2.2	3.9 2.1	4.5 2.5
C72	Malignant neoplasm of spinal cord, cranial nerves and other parts of central nervous system	M F	0.2 0.2	0.7 -	0.6 0.4	0.3 0.1	0.2 0.4	0.1 0.1	0.1 0.2	0.2 0.1	0.1 -	0.1 0.2
C73	Malignant neoplasm of thyroid gland	M F	1.3 3.4	- -	- -	0.1 0.1	0.2 0.6	0.3 0.5	0.7 1.4	0.8 4.3	0.9 3.5	1.1 4.6
C74	Malignant neoplasm of adrenal gland	M F	0.3 0.4	2.5 3.3	0.7 0.8	0.3 0.2	0.1 0.1	0.1 0.1	- -	- 0.1	0.1 0.1	0.1 0.2
C75	Malignant neoplasm of other endocrine glands and related structures	M F	0.2 0.1	0.4 -	0.1 0.2	0.1 0.1	0.2 0.1	0.1 -	0.3 0.1	0.1 0.1	0.1 -	0.2 0.1

40-44	45-49	50-54	55-59	60-64	65-69	70-74	75-79	80-84	85 and over		Site description	ICD (10th Revision) number
1.2	1.5	2.6	2.7	4.2	5.8	7.0	8.0	11.4	15.4	M	Malignant neoplasm of other connective and soft tissue	C49
1.4	1.9	2.0	2.5	2.6	3.1	4.1	5.7	6.8	6.7	F		
0.1	0.6	0.9	1.9	2.2	2.9	5.9	3.6	7.2	8.6	M	Malignant neoplasm of breast	C50
113.7	176.5	276.1	295.7	315.9	270.9	306.0	343.9	351.9	419.8	F		
1.9	2.7	3.1	2.7	4.8	7.0	11.2	12.7	17.5	24.0	F	Malignant neoplasm of vulva	C51
0.3	0.3	1.0	0.7	1.4	1.3	1.3	3.1	2.8	3.9	F	Malignant neoplasm of vagina	C52
16.3	14.5	10.8	10.6	11.2	12.8	14.5	18.5	16.1	11.9	F	Malignant neoplasm of cervix uteri	C53
4.7	10.2	25.0	44.8	60.6	60.7	56.8	57.0	57.0	51.1	F	Malignant neoplasm of corpus uteri	C54
0.5	0.7	1.1	1.8	2.5	2.1	2.4	4.2	4.0	8.5	F	Malignant neoplasm of uterus, part unspecified	C55
10.0	21.6	31.9	44.1	54.8	61.4	66.8	73.4	73.9	62.7	F	Malignant neoplasm of ovary and other unspecified female genital organs	C56-C57
9.9	21.5	31.1	43.1	53.8	60.1	66.0	71.8	72.8	61.5	F	Malignant neoplasm of ovary	C56
0.1	0.1	0.8	1.0	1.0	1.2	0.8	1.6	1.1	1.2	F	Malignant neoplasm of other and unspecified female genital organs	C57
-	-	-	-	-	-	-	-	-	-	F	Malignant neoplasm of placenta	C58
1.2	1.3	1.3	2.5	3.7	2.8	5.5	7.1	6.5	8.6	M	Malignant neoplasm of penis	C60
1.0	7.1	33.4	102.6	239.0	442.4	598.8	753.4	814.3	984.0	M	Malignant neoplasm of prostate	C61
12.3	8.9	5.6	3.9	2.3	1.5	1.8	1.7	1.7	1.9	M	Malignant neoplasm of testis	C62
-	0.3	0.1	0.2	0.5	0.8	1.2	1.2	0.7	2.2	M	Malignant neoplasm of other and unspecified male genital organs	C63
4.6	7.8	14.5	19.1	27.2	39.7	44.6	54.6	55.1	63.0	M	Malignant neoplasm of kidney, except renal pelvis	C64
2.0	3.8	7.4	9.7	13.5	20.1	19.5	25.8	25.9	26.6	F		
0.4	0.4	0.5	1.1	2.5	4.1	4.3	4.7	2.9	4.5	M	Malignant neoplasm of renal pelvis	C65
0.1	0.3	0.1	0.8	1.1	1.2	2.0	2.0	2.7	2.3	F		
-	0.1	0.3	0.7	1.9	2.3	3.8	5.5	6.0	2.2	M	Malignant neoplasm of ureter	C66
0.1	0.1	0.2	0.2	0.6	1.0	2.3	2.4	0.7	1.9	F		
2.8	5.5	13.2	27.7	52.5	82.6	126.1	183.5	212.8	298.3	M	Malignant neoplasm of bladder	C67
1.2	2.3	4.1	7.8	14.1	21.9	34.4	49.3	63.1	80.3	F		
-	0.1	0.1	0.4	0.8	1.3	1.5	2.3	3.6	3.0	M	Malignant neoplasm of other and unspecified urinery organs	C68
0.1	-	0.1	0.1	0.2	0.2	0.4	0.3	-	1.6	F		
0.3	0.6	1.1	1.2	2.2	2.0	2.4	2.8	2.7	2.2	M	Malignant neoplasm of eye and adnexa	C69
0.1	0.4	0.7	1.2	1.1	2.1	1.3	2.3	1.7	1.7	F		
-	0.1	0.1	0.1	0.1	0.5	0.5	0.1	0.2	0.7	M	Malignant neoplasm of meninges	C70
0.2	0.2	0.1	0.3	0.3	0.4	0.5	0.6	1.1	1.2	F		
5.0	7.7	11.2	14.2	18.3	24.6	25.7	28.2	23.9	15.0	M	Malignant neoplasm of brain	C71
4.1	4.9	5.7	8.8	12.2	15.6	18.1	16.0	14.4	12.3	F		
0.1	0.3	0.2	0.2	0.3	0.3	0.2	0.6	0.5	0.4	M	Malignant neoplasm of spinal cord, cranial nerves and other parts of central nervous system	C72
0.1	0.1	0.3	0.2	0.4	0.1	0.4	0.1	0.7	0.1	F		
1.3	1.6	1.3	2.3	2.1	3.2	2.8	3.9	5.6	4.1	M	Malignant neoplasm of thyroid gland	C73
4.1	4.0	5.4	4.6	5.0	3.9	5.8	4.7	5.4	6.9	F		
0.1	0.3	0.5	0.1	0.5	0.6	0.5	1.7	1.4	0.4	M	Malignant neoplasm of adrenal gland	C74
0.2	0.5	0.3	0.7	0.7	0.9	0.4	1.3	0.4	0.1	F		
0.1	0.1	0.1	0.1	0.3	0.3	0.6	0.4	-	0.4	M	Malignant neoplasm of other endocrine glands and related structures	C75
0.2	-	0.2	0.1	0.5	0.1	0.6	0.1	0.1	0.1	F		

Table 3 Series MB1 no. 32

Table 3   Rates per 100,000 population - *continued*

ICD (10th Revision) number	Site description		All ages	Under 1	1-4	5-9	10-14	15-19	20-24	25-29	30-34	35-39
C76	Malignant neoplasm of other and ill-defined sites	M F	0.9 1.3	0.7 0.4	0.2 0.1	0.1 0.1	0.1 0.3	0.2 -	0.1 0.1	0.2 0.1	0.5 0.2	0.3 0.4
C77	Secondary and unspecified malignant neoplasm of lymph nodes	M F	1.5 1.1	- -	- -	0.1 0.1	- -	- 0.1	- 0.1	0.1 0.1	0.3 0.1	0.5 0.4
C78	Secondary malignant neoplasm of respiratory and digestive organs	M F	7.9 8.7	- -	- -	- -	- -	0.1 -	- 0.1	0.1 0.2	0.3 0.6	0.6 0.8
C79	Secondary malignant neoplasm of other sites	M F	3.7 3.5	- -	0.1 -	- 0.1	0.1 -	0.1 0.1	- -	0.1 0.2	0.2 0.2	0.3 0.3
C80	Malignant neoplasm without specification of site	M F	9.5 12.0	- -	- 0.1	- -	- -	0.1 0.1	0.3 0.1	0.2 0.2	0.6 0.4	0.6 0.8
C81	Hodgkin's disease	M F	2.8 2.0	- -	0.2 0.2	0.6 0.3	0.8 1.3	2.6 2.6	5.2 3.4	3.9 3.7	3.4 2.9	3.7 2.2
C82-C85	Non-Hodgkin's lymphoma	M F	17.2 14.4	0.7 -	0.7 0.4	1.1 0.3	1.0 0.6	2.2 1.5	2.0 1.7	2.4 2.6	5.0 3.1	5.9 4.1
C82	Follicular (nodular) non-Hodgkin's lymphoma	M F	2.2 2.2	- -	- -	- -	0.1 -	0.1 -	- 0.1	0.3 0.2	0.9 0.7	0.9 0.6
C83	Diffuse non-Hodgkin's lymphoma	M F	6.2 4.7	0.7 -	0.5 0.3	0.5 0.3	0.5 0.1	1.0 1.2	0.9 0.7	1.2 0.7	1.6 0.7	2.3 1.5
C84	Peripheral and cutaneous T-cell lymphomas	M F	1.1 0.7	- -	0.1 -	- -	- 0.1	0.4 -	0.1 -	0.2 0.1	0.5 0.4	0.5 0.5
C85	Other and unspecified types on non-Hodgkin's lymphoma	M F	7.7 6.8	- -	0.2 0.1	0.6 -	0.5 0.4	0.8 0.3	0.9 0.8	0.8 1.3	2.0 1.2	2.2 1.5
C88	Malignant immunoproliferative diseases	M F	0.6 0.3	- -	0.1 -	- -	- -	- -	- -	- -	- -	- -
C90	Multiple myeloma and malignant plasma cell neoplasms	M F	6.3 5.3	- -	- -	- -	- -	- -	- -	- 0.1	0.2 0.1	0.4 0.5
C91-C95	All leukaemias	M F	13.1 9.7	3.9 4.8	6.9 6.6	3.1 3.2	2.7 2.5	2.6 1.4	3.0 1.5	2.5 2.2	2.6 1.7	4.0 1.9
C91	Lymphoid leukaemia	M F	6.8 4.6	1.4 2.9	5.9 5.6	2.6 2.6	2.1 1.5	1.4 0.5	0.7 0.8	0.7 0.6	0.7 0.3	1.2 0.5
C92	Myeloid leukaemia	M F	5.7 4.5	2.5 1.5	0.9 0.9	0.5 0.6	0.6 1.0	1.0 0.9	1.9 0.7	1.6 1.4	1.8 1.3	2.7 1.3
C93	Monocytic leukaemia	M F	0.2 0.2	- 0.4	0.1 -	0.1 -	- -	0.1 -	0.1 -	0.1 0.1	0.1 0.1	0.1 0.1
C94	Other leukaemias of specified cell type	M F	0.1 0.0	- -	- -	- -	- -	- -	0.1 -	0.1 -	- -	- -
C95	Leukaemia of unspecified cell type	M F	0.4 0.4	- -	- 0.2	- -	- -	0.1 0.1	0.1 -	0.1 -	- -	- 0.1
C96	Other and unspecified malignant neoplasms of lymphoid, haematopoietic and related tissue	M F	0.1 0.1	- -	0.2 0.1	0.1 0.1	- -	- -	- -	- -	- 0.1	0.2 -
C97	Malignant neoplasms of independent (primary) multiple sites	M F	- -	- -	- -	- -	- -	- -	- -	- -	- -	- -
D00	Carcinoma in situ of oral cavity, oesophagus and stomach	M F	0.5 0.3	- -	- -	- -	- -	- 0.1	- 0.1	- -	- -	- -
D01	Carcinoma in situ of other and unspecified digestive organs	M F	0.8 0.7	- -	- -	- -	- -	0.1 -	- -	0.2 0.1	0.1 0.1	0.2 0.3
D02	Carcinoma in situ of middle ear and respiratory system	M F	0.7 0.2	- -	- -	- -	- -	- -	- -	- -	0.1 -	- -
D03	Melanoma in situ	M F	3.1 4.4	- -	- -	- -	- 0.1	0.3 0.3	0.3 1.1	1.0 1.6	0.9 2.0	1.3 2.8

40-44	45-49	50-54	55-59	60-64	65-69	70-74	75-79	80-84	85 and over		Site description	ICD (10th Revision) number
0.2	0.4	0.5	1.1	1.1	1.4	3.2	3.3	7.7	12.0	M	Malignant neoplasm of other and	C76
0.5	0.7	1.1	0.8	0.8	2.3	3.8	4.5	6.4	13.3	F	ill-defined sites	
1.0	1.5	1.7	2.1	4.1	5.4	5.4	7.1	7.0	7.5	M	Secondary and unspecified malignant	C77
0.8	0.4	0.9	2.2	2.5	2.9	3.8	3.6	4.0	5.5	F	neoplasm of lymph nodes	
1.7	1.8	4.7	8.3	16.5	21.3	37.9	55.7	67.4	80.9	M	Secondary malignant neoplasm of	C78
1.3	3.0	4.4	7.6	12.5	18.6	31.5	42.2	52.9	62.5	F	respiratory and digestive organs	
0.7	1.2	2.6	4.4	7.2	11.0	17.2	22.8	33.3	34.5	M	Secondary malignant neoplasm of	C79
0.4	1.8	2.2	4.1	5.8	10.1	13.7	17.1	16.9	18.2	F	other sites	
1.4	2.3	5.3	8.6	14.8	26.0	41.8	68.3	89.8	128.5	M	Malignant neoplasm without	C80
1.8	2.7	4.4	9.2	14.9	24.6	38.8	52.5	75.8	119.5	F	specification of site	
2.9	2.7	2.7	3.1	3.1	2.9	3.4	3.3	3.1	3.0	M	Hodgkin's disease	C81
1.9	1.2	0.8	1.7	2.8	3.1	2.5	2.0	2.0	1.7	F		
9.1	13.3	20.5	29.0	38.6	52.3	62.0	74.5	84.3	98.9	M	Non-Hodgkin's lymphoma	C82-C85
6.9	8.6	14.9	21.1	29.2	35.1	44.0	57.0	61.7	57.2	F		
1.8	3.2	4.1	5.3	6.0	5.7	5.5	6.3	5.8	4.9	M	Follicular (nodular) non-Hodgkin's	C82
1.8	2.5	4.0	5.2	6.5	5.6	4.8	6.6	5.8	2.3	F	lymphoma	
3.0	4.0	8.1	10.1	13.1	19.8	25.2	25.3	27.0	29.6	M	Diffuse non-Hodgkin's lymphoma	C83
2.1	2.5	4.1	6.6	9.3	11.0	17.0	20.5	19.1	16.9	F	lymphoma	
0.9	0.7	1.6	2.2	2.3	3.4	2.9	4.2	5.8	6.7	M	Peripheral and cutaneous T-cell	C84
0.5	0.5	0.8	1.3	1.3	2.3	1.4	1.7	1.4	2.6	F	lymphomas	
3.4	5.5	6.7	11.4	17.3	23.4	28.4	38.7	45.6	57.7	M	Other and unspecified types on non-	C85
2.4	3.1	6.0	8.1	12.2	16.1	20.7	28.2	35.4	35.3	F	Hodgkin's lymphoma	
-	0.1	0.4	0.6	0.8	1.4	2.6	4.1	4.8	8.2	M	Malignant immunoproliferative	C88
0.1	0.1	0.1	0.2	0.3	0.4	1.0	1.8	2.0	2.3	F	diseases	
1.7	2.5	4.4	8.9	14.6	22.4	29.8	36.5	49.0	48.0	M	Multiple myeloma and malignant	C90
1.0	1.7	3.2	6.1	9.5	13.9	17.0	24.1	31.7	33.0	F	plasma cell neoplasms	
3.6	6.1	10.4	14.8	24.9	34.9	45.0	69.4	76.1	124.4	M	All leukaemias	C91-C95
2.6	4.3	6.7	10.2	10.8	18.9	27.9	35.7	45.1	64.4	F		
1.4	2.7	4.7	9.0	13.9	19.8	23.6	33.8	36.0	63.7	M	Lymphoid leukaemia	C91
0.7	1.8	2.3	4.3	5.0	9.6	12.9	16.8	22.3	31.8	F		
2.0	3.1	5.2	5.0	10.1	13.7	19.0	32.6	34.3	52.8	M	Myeloid leukaemia	C92
1.8	2.2	4.1	5.5	5.3	8.6	13.7	16.5	19.1	26.9	F		
0.1	0.1	0.2	0.2	0.3	0.6	0.5	0.7	1.2	0.4	M	Monocytic leukaemia	C93
0.1	0.1	0.2	0.1	0.1	0.3	0.2	0.8	0.3	1.4	F		
0.1	-	0.1	0.1	0.3	0.1	0.6	-	0.7	-	M	Other leukaemias of specified cell	C94
-	0.1	0.1	-	-	0.1	0.4	0.1	0.1	0.3	F	type	
0.1	0.1	0.2	0.4	0.4	0.8	1.4	2.3	3.9	7.5	M	Leukaemia of unspecified cell type	C95
-	0.1	0.1	0.2	0.3	0.4	0.7	1.5	3.3	3.9	F		
-	-	-	0.1	0.2	-	0.3	0.4	-	1.1	M	Other and unspecified malignant	C96
-	0.1	-	0.1	-	0.3	0.1	0.3	0.1	0.3	F	neoplasms of lymphoid, haematopoietic and related tissue	
-	-	-	-	-	-	-	-	-	-	M	Malignant neoplasms of independent	C97
-	-	-	-	-	-	-	-	-	-	F	(primary) multiple sites	
0.1	0.3	0.5	0.6	1.5	1.3	1.9	3.5	2.9	0.7	M	Carcinoma in situ of oral cavity,	D00
0.1	0.1	0.1	0.6	0.2	0.8	0.7	2.3	2.0	2.5	F	oesophagus and stomach	
0.3	0.5	0.1	1.4	1.6	2.8	4.2	4.1	6.5	4.5	M	Carcinoma in situ of other and	D01
0.2	0.5	0.4	1.3	1.5	1.8	2.1	2.9	3.1	3.2	F	unspecified digestive organs	
0.1	0.2	1.0	1.2	2.0	2.5	2.8	4.4	4.1	0.7	M	Carcinoma in situ of middle ear and	D02
-	0.1	0.4	0.5	0.7	0.4	0.8	0.8	0.3	0.4	F	respiratory system	
1.8	2.1	3.8	5.3	6.8	9.2	12.4	14.3	14.7	18.0	M	Melanoma in situ	D03
4.1	4.7	6.3	6.8	8.0	10.7	12.1	10.6	13.8	11.0	F		

Table 3   Rates per 100,000 population - *continued*

ICD (10th Revision) number	Site description		All ages	Under 1	1-4	5-9	10-14	15-19	20-24	25-29	30-34	35-39
D04	Carcinoma in situ of skin	M F	7.8 14.8	- -	- -	- -	- -	- -	- -	- 0.2	0.3 0.3	0.8 0.5
D05	Carcinoma in situ of breast	M F	0.1 12.0	- -	- -	- -	- -	- -	- -	- 0.8	- 1.5	- 4.0
D06	Carcinoma in situ of cervix uteri	F	77.3	-	-	-	-	14.7	231.8	311.4	238.4	143.3
D07	Carcinoma in situ of other and unspecified genital organs	M F	1.7 2.4	- -	- -	- -	- -	- 0.2	0.3 0.6	0.2 1.1	0.3 2.3	0.4 3.9
D09	Carcinoma in situ of other and unspecified sites	M F	9.3 3.1	- -	- -	- -	- -	- -	0.3 0.1	0.1 0.1	0.5 0.1	1.1 0.2
D33	Benign neoplasm of brain and other parts of central nervous system	M F	1.0 1.0	- -	0.1 0.3	0.1 -	0.2 0.2	0.3 0.5	0.3 0.5	0.5 0.4	0.9 0.5	1.2 1.3
D35.2	Benign neoplasm of pituitary gland	M F	0.8 0.6	- -	- -	- -	0.1 0.1	0.1 -	0.2 0.2	0.2 0.4	0.6 1.0	0.5 0.5
D35.3	Benign neoplasm of craniopharyngeal duct	M F	- -	- -	- -	- -	- -	- -	- -	- -	- -	- -
D35.4	Benign neoplasm of pineal gland	M F	- -	- -	- -	- -	- -	- -	- -	- -	- -	- -
D37	Neoplasm of uncertain or unknown behaviour of oral cavity and digestive organs	M F	2.7 2.7	- 0.4	- -	- -	0.3 0.8	0.4 1.1	0.4 0.7	0.3 0.7	0.3 0.9	0.7 0.7
D38	Neoplasm of uncertain or unknown behaviour of middle ear and respiratory and intrathoracic organs	M F	0.3 0.3	- -	- 0.2	- -	- -	- -	- -	0.1 -	0.1 0.1	0.2 0.1
D39	Neoplasm of uncertain or unknown behaviour of female genital organs	F	1.2	-	0.1	0.1	0.4	0.6	0.7	1.4	1.1	1.4
D40	Neoplasm of uncertain or unknown behaviour of male genital organs	M	0.4	0.7	0.2	0.1	-	0.1	0.3	0.5	0.2	0.4
D41	Neoplasm of uncertain or unknown behaviour of urinary organs	M F	7.7 3.0	0.4 -	- -	- -	- -	- -	0.1 -	0.8 0.1	0.5 0.3	0.7 0.4
D42	Neoplasm of uncertain or unknown behaviour of meninges	M F	0.1 0.1	- -	- -	- 0.1	- -	- -	0.1 0.1	- -	- -	- 0.2
D43	Neoplasm of uncertain or unknown behaviour of brain and central nervous system	M F	1.1 1.0	0.7 -	0.1 0.1	0.3 0.3	0.3 0.3	0.3 0.3	0.1 0.2	0.7 0.1	0.5 0.1	0.4 1.0
D44	Neoplasm of uncertain or unknown behaviour of endocrine glands	M F	0.4 0.4	- -	0.1 0.1	0.2 0.2	0.1 0.1	0.2 0.4	0.3 0.2	0.1 0.2	0.1 0.3	0.4 0.5
D45	Polycythaemia vera	M F	0.8 0.6	- -	- -	- -	- -	0.1 -	- -	0.1 0.1	0.3 0.1	0.2 0.2
D46	Myelodysplastic syndromes	M F	4.6 4.0	- -	0.1 0.1	- 0.1	0.1 -	- 0.2	0.1 0.2	0.1 0.2	0.1 0.2	0.2 0.1
D47	Other neoplasms of uncertain or unknown behaviour of lymphoid, haematopoietic and related tissue	M F	3.6 4.0	0.4 -	- -	0.1 -	0.1 0.1	- 0.1	0.1 0.3	0.2 0.5	0.2 0.3	0.6 1.0
D48	Neoplasm of uncertain or unknown behaviour of other and unspecified sites	M F	1.0 1.5	2.8 0.7	- 0.2	0.1 0.3	0.2 0.3	0.3 0.6	0.7 1.3	0.4 0.8	0.6 1.0	0.8 1.2
O01	Hydatidiform mole	F	1.0	-	-	-	-	1.6	2.3	3.7	3.1	1.9

40-44	45-49	50-54	55-59	60-64	65-69	70-74	75-79	80-84	85 and over		Site description	ICD (10th Revision) number
1.3	2.2	4.4	9.3	14.8	23.8	36.6	52.5	72.9	73.8	M	Carcinoma in situ of skin	D04
1.3	3.0	5.3	10.4	20.7	40.4	53.9	73.7	94.5	111.3	F		
0.1	0.1	0.1	0.1	-	0.1	0.6	0.3	0.5	0.7	M	Carcinoma in situ of breast	D05
7.7	16.4	46.3	40.6	41.8	20.0	16.7	13.3	8.8	6.4	F		
80.6	47.2	27.7	20.0	17.8	7.3	2.7	2.0	1.8	0.9	F	Carcinoma in situ of cervix uteri	D06
0.3	0.5	1.2	2.0	4.9	9.7	10.4	7.1	4.1	2.6	M	Carcinoma in situ of other and unspecified genital organs	D07
3.9	4.5	4.5	3.7	3.9	3.1	3.3	4.5	1.7	2.7	F		
1.4	3.7	5.3	12.5	20.3	32.3	47.1	64.8	65.7	56.6	M	Carcinoma in situ of other and unspecified sites	D09
0.7	1.0	2.9	4.1	6.0	9.2	13.7	13.9	14.6	12.6	F		
1.4	2.3	1.6	1.9	0.9	1.8	1.6	1.7	0.2	0.7	M	Benign neoplasm of brain and other parts of central nervous system	D33
1.2	1.2	1.6	1.9	2.1	1.8	2.2	1.4	0.6	0.9	F		
0.6	1.4	1.4	1.3	1.6	2.7	2.9	2.2	2.7	0.7	M	Benign neoplasm of pituitary gland	D35.2
0.7	0.8	0.8	1.1	1.4	1.8	1.0	1.2	0.6	0.3	F		
-	-	-	-	-	-	-	-	-	-	M	Benign neoplasm of craniopharyngeal duct	D35.3
-	-	-	-	-	-	-	-	-	-	F		
-	-	-	-	-	-	-	-	-	-	M	Benign neoplasm of pineal gland	D35.4
-	-	-	-	-	-	-	-	-	-	F		
0.4	1.0	2.5	3.6	6.4	9.0	14.0	15.1	13.0	18.4	M	Neoplasm of uncertain or unknown behaviour of oral cavity and digestive organs	D37
1.5	1.5	2.0	2.6	4.9	6.9	7.8	10.2	11.8	12.4	F		
-	0.3	0.2	0.3	0.5	0.6	1.4	2.2	1.4	3.4	M	Neoplasm of uncertain or unknown behaviour of middle ear and respiratory and intrathoracic organs	D38
0.1	0.2	0.1	0.3	0.3	1.0	1.5	0.9	0.9	1.2	F		
1.4	2.5	1.8	1.5	1.9	1.4	1.9	1.2	1.4	1.2	F	Neoplasm of uncertain or unknown behaviour of female genital organs	D39
0.3	0.3	0.5	0.6	0.2	0.6	1.1	1.0	0.7	1.9	M	Neoplasm of uncertain or unknown behaviour of male genital organs	D40
2.0	3.0	6.4	11.0	18.6	28.5	34.6	43.7	53.9	50.6	M	Neoplasm of uncertain or unknown behaviour of urinary organs	D41
0.7	1.0	2.7	3.8	6.9	7.0	14.2	11.7	13.4	12.2	F		
0.1	0.1	0.2	0.1	0.2	0.1	0.1	0.4	0.2	-	M	Neoplasm of uncertain or unknown behaviour of meninges	D42
0.1	0.1	-	0.1	0.1	0.4	0.4	0.2	-	0.1	F		
1.1	0.6	0.8	0.8	1.9	1.5	3.4	4.9	7.7	10.1	M	Neoplasm of uncertain or unknown behaviour of brain and central nervous system	D43
0.6	0.6	0.2	1.0	1.0	1.1	3.7	4.0	5.4	4.8	F		
0.2	0.5	0.3	0.7	0.7	0.9	0.8	1.2	1.0	2.2	M	Neoplasm of uncertain or unknown behaviour of endocrine glands	D44
0.3	0.3	0.2	0.4	0.9	0.5	0.7	1.3	0.7	1.3	F		
0.7	0.4	0.5	1.5	2.4	2.3	2.6	5.7	4.3	3.4	M	Polycythaemia vera	D45
0.3	0.2	0.8	0.8	0.9	2.1	1.8	2.6	2.7	2.7	F		
0.4	0.5	1.0	2.5	3.9	9.4	17.8	34.8	52.9	100.1	M	Myelodysplastic syndromes	D46
0.5	0.4	1.0	1.5	2.6	6.2	8.7	17.6	29.9	52.7	F		
1.0	1.9	2.6	4.9	7.8	9.2	14.6	22.6	30.4	33.0	M	Other neoplasms of uncertain or unknown behaviour of lymphoid, haematopoietic and related tissue	D47
1.3	1.8	3.4	2.9	5.3	8.5	13.9	19.6	21.0	25.3	F		
0.9	1.2	0.9	1.4	1.2	1.6	2.1	3.9	2.9	8.2	M	Neoplasm of uncertain or unknown behaviour of other and unspecified sites	D48
1.4	1.6	2.2	2.4	1.6	2.3	1.3	3.0	3.6	4.6	F		
0.6	0.4	0.4	-	-	-	-	-	-	-	F	Hydatidiform mole	O01

Table 4 Series MB1 no. 32

Table 4 Registrations of newly diagnosed cases of cancer: site, sex and government office for the region of residence, 2001

**England, government offices for the regions
Registered by May 2004**

ICD (10th Revision) number	Site description		England	North East	North West	Yorkshire and the Humber	East Midlands	West Midlands	East of England	London	South East	South West
	All registrations	M	151,069	9,116	22,472	16,562	13,109	16,550	15,340	14,259	23,845	19,816
		F	170,127	10,407	25,735	18,752	14,902	18,615	17,109	16,451	26,463	21,693
C00-C97	All cancers	M	139,387	8,414	20,783	15,146	12,001	15,321	14,182	13,351	21,905	18,284
		F	135,657	8,065	20,498	14,859	11,614	14,542	13,751	13,152	21,416	17,760
C00-C97 xC44	All cancers excluding nmsc	M	112,516	6,698	16,347	11,908	9,328	11,970	11,812	12,806	18,289	13,358
		F	112,134	6,436	16,186	11,941	9,448	11,583	11,885	12,801	18,383	13,471
C00-C14	Malignant neoplasm of lip, mouth and pharynx	M	2,606	164	451	275	209	275	244	323	406	259
		F	1,461	73	229	168	126	161	130	193	222	159
C00	Malignant neoplasm of lip	M	159	15	21	28	12	15	20	5	29	14
		F	79	12	8	15	3	4	10	7	16	4
C01	Malignant neoplasm of base of tongue	M	184	13	30	21	22	19	19	23	20	17
		F	63	3	12	7	3	9	8	9	8	4
C02	Malignant neoplasm of other and unspecified parts of tongue	M	443	26	72	46	35	41	38	59	73	53
		F	301	5	40	35	26	39	31	44	51	30
C03	Malignant neoplasm of gum	M	106	1	11	5	12	9	22	19	19	8
		F	88	2	12	7	13	12	9	11	13	9
C04	Malignant neoplasm of floor of mouth	M	241	22	59	25	16	26	16	25	37	15
		F	106	5	21	9	12	11	9	13	14	12
C05	Malignant neoplasm of palate	M	119	8	26	8	11	12	7	13	17	17
		F	104	11	14	14	10	6	8	9	16	16
C06	Malignant neoplasm of other and unspecified parts of mouth	M	199	8	42	31	14	12	15	29	28	20
		F	149	6	28	15	16	13	9	22	27	13
C07	Malignant neoplasm of parotid gland	M	199	9	19	25	12	20	19	26	48	21
		F	145	10	17	23	13	17	12	21	14	18
C08	Malignant neoplasm of other and unspecified major salivary glands	M	55	2	7	5	7	6	3	7	11	7
		F	50	3	7	2	6	8	4	6	7	7
C09	Malignant neoplasm of tonsil	M	332	23	60	27	15	39	40	42	49	37
		F	117	7	19	12	5	20	8	12	18	16
C10	Malignant neoplasm of oropharynx	M	104	8	20	10	14	17	6	10	13	6
		F	29	1	5	3	3	2	4	4	4	3
C11	Malignant neoplasm of nasopharynx	M	107	4	10	6	12	12	14	16	12	21
		F	64	-	15	5	3	9	3	11	7	11
C12	Malignant neoplasm of piriform sinus	M	165	14	30	19	10	28	16	19	22	7
		F	36	3	7	2	3	5	3	5	5	3
C13	Malignant neoplasm of hypopharynx	M	78	7	17	11	4	11	3	9	12	4
		F	69	5	14	9	7	4	8	7	8	7
C14	Malignant neoplasm of other and ill-defined sites in the lip, oral cavity and pharynx	M	115	4	27	8	13	8	6	21	16	12
		F	61	-	10	10	3	2	4	12	14	6
C15	Malignant neoplasm of oesophagus	M	3,806	166	628	364	377	417	358	380	637	479
		F	2,274	124	366	226	206	260	207	242	378	265
C16	Malignant neoplasm of stomach	M	4,741	323	790	518	431	572	495	554	606	452
		F	2,626	213	430	338	226	289	247	298	337	248
C17	Malignant neoplasm of small intestine	M	316	18	46	33	17	43	30	34	51	44
		F	275	11	41	30	23	26	31	25	44	44
C18-C20	Malignant neoplasm of colon and rectum	M	14,836	973	2,245	1,583	1,251	1,725	1,561	1,553	2,227	1,718
		F	12,693	734	1,781	1,341	1,018	1,275	1,413	1,341	2,159	1,631
C18	Malignant neoplasm of colon	M	8,858	538	1,335	886	727	1,010	892	946	1,356	1,168
		F	8,677	481	1,223	852	702	872	917	899	1,510	1,221
C19	Malignant neoplasm of rectosigmoid junction	M	1,205	108	194	163	106	101	140	132	185	76
		F	846	64	115	125	62	74	119	108	119	60

Table 4 Registrations in government offices for the regions - *continued*

ICD (10th Revision) number	Site description		England	North East	North West	Yorkshire and the Humber	East Midlands	West Midlands	East of England	London	South East	South West
C20	Malignant neoplasm of rectum	M F	4,773 3,170	327 189	716 443	534 364	418 254	614 329	529 377	475 334	686 530	474 350
C21	Malignant neoplasm of anus and anal canal	M F	255 385	18 21	34 59	32 28	21 25	19 40	14 26	53 51	38 73	26 62
C22	Malignant neoplasm of liver and intrahepatic bile ducts	M F	1,242 883	79 61	225 227	121 75	93 77	116 82	92 64	198 119	183 94	135 84
C23	Malignant neoplasm of gallbladder	M F	124 287	14 13	8 42	17 43	14 21	14 27	13 26	16 34	19 52	9 29
C24	Malignant neoplasm of other and unspecified parts of biliary tract	M F	291 307	17 17	33 26	21 31	22 17	27 30	29 36	40 36	62 62	40 52
C25	Malignant neoplasm of pancreas	M F	2,807 2,986	162 171	368 380	289 344	275 252	281 296	275 355	349 385	451 482	357 321
C26	Malignant neoplasm of other and ill-defined digestive organs	M F	230 327	3 2	37 39	15 14	23 20	11 15	11 32	36 51	54 86	40 68
C30	Malignant neoplasm of nasal cavity and middle ear	M F	100 88	9 6	12 14	8 7	5 3	6 7	16 8	12 6	23 24	9 13
C31	Malignant neoplasm of accessory sinuses	M F	90 54	4 2	14 12	10 -	6 2	8 9	8 4	12 9	16 9	12 7
C32	Malignant neoplasm of larynx	M F	1,477 328	117 26	259 61	178 38	120 29	173 28	137 32	161 50	207 41	125 23
C33-C34	Malignant neoplasm of trachea, bronchus and lung	M F	18,577 11,963	1,380 976	2,984 2,129	2,136 1,475	1,564 971	1,972 1,133	1,775 1,110	2,295 1,439	2,653 1,645	1,818 1,085
C33	Malignant neoplasm of trachea	M F	32 23	1 1	10 9	2 2	4 1	4 1	2 3	1 2	7 2	1 2
C34	Malignant neoplasm of bronchus and lung	M F	18,545 11,940	1,379 975	2,974 2,120	2,134 1,473	1,560 970	1,968 1,132	1,773 1,107	2,294 1,437	2,646 1,643	1,817 1,083
C37	Malignant neoplasm of thymus	M F	30 30	2 3	1 3	7 2	4 3	3 5	2 4	2 4	4 1	5 5
C38	Malignant neoplasm of heart, mediastinum and pleura	M F	136 97	6 1	29 23	13 11	9 6	10 4	7 6	7 12	24 15	31 19
C39	Malignant neoplasm of other and ill-defined sites in the respiratory system and intrathoracic organs	M F	4 3	- -	- 1	- -	- -	- -	- 1	3 1	- -	1 -
C40	Malignant neoplasm of bone and articular cartilage of limbs	M F	112 90	8 6	17 8	8 10	11 4	15 13	10 6	17 13	15 14	11 16
C41	Malignant neoplasm of bone and articular cartilage of other and unspecified sites	M F	111 117	6 2	26 36	7 6	8 11	6 10	15 12	11 9	15 15	17 16
C43	Malignant melanoma of skin	M F	2,638 3,424	105 188	282 424	255 358	189 261	281 320	286 371	230 278	538 647	472 577
C44	Other malignant neoplasms of skin	M F	26,871 23,523	1,716 1,629	4,436 4,312	3,238 2,918	2,673 2,166	3,351 2,959	2,370 1,866	545 351	3,616 3,033	4,926 4,289
C45	Mesothelioma	M F	1,423 329	116 22	222 37	146 33	95 26	118 27	166 41	137 43	267 68	156 32
C46	Kaposi's sarcoma	M F	63 17	1 -	4 -	1 2	2 -	8 -	4 1	32 14	8 -	3 -
C47	Malignant neoplasm of peripheral nerves and autonomic nervous system	M F	39 48	4 4	2 5	4 6	6 5	6 6	3 3	3 4	4 9	7 6
C48	Malignant neoplasm of retroperitoneum and peritoneum	M F	97 183	3 20	17 23	8 15	7 24	11 19	9 20	10 23	20 20	12 19

Table 4 Registrations in government offices for the regions - continued

ICD (10th Revision) number	Site description	Sex	England	North East	North West	Yorkshire and the Humber	East Midlands	West Midlands	East of England	London	South East	South West
C49	Malignant neoplasm of other connective and soft tissue	M	536	26	76	64	49	53	51	40	77	100
		F	469	16	57	54	44	55	51	39	73	80
C50	Malignant neoplasm of breast	M	245	16	29	14	6	34	30	37	45	34
		F	34,347	1,715	4,792	3,346	2,874	3,688	3,793	4,009	5,911	4,219
C51	Malignant neoplasm of vulva	F	866	67	133	85	88	105	82	66	125	115
C52	Malignant neoplasm of vagina	F	166	12	31	18	17	18	13	16	27	14
C53	Malignant neoplasm of cervix uteri	F	2,418	152	403	303	218	306	193	273	292	278
C54	Malignant neoplasm of corpus uteri	F	4,678	198	626	438	477	527	572	507	712	621
C55	Malignant neoplasm of uterus, part unspecified	F	276	20	50	44	24	31	24	26	38	19
C56-C57	Malignant neoplasm of ovary and other unspecified female genital organs	F	5,735	310	737	631	489	639	636	600	1,015	678
C56	Malignant neoplasm of ovary	F	5,635	308	727	626	483	625	628	586	994	658
C57	Malignant neoplasm of other and unspecified female genital organs	F	100	2	10	5	6	14	8	14	21	20
C58	Malignant neoplasm of placenta	F	6	-	1	-	-	1	2	1	1	-
C60	Malignant neoplasm of penis	M	332	21	45	48	32	37	40	26	43	40
C61	Malignant neoplasm of prostate	M	26,027	1,382	3,463	2,534	1,938	2,938	3,027	2,895	4,534	3,316
C62	Malignant neoplasm of testis	M	1,653	90	194	181	134	159	162	218	303	212
C63	Malignant neoplasm of other and unspecified male genital organs	M	54	3	9	4	8	10	7	5	3	5
C64	Malignant neoplasm of kidney, except renal pelvis	M	2,701	168	342	298	259	278	256	281	477	342
		F	1,648	106	245	230	119	136	187	192	249	184
C65	Malignant neoplasm of renal pelvis	M	203	25	27	38	19	18	16	13	35	12
		F	121	6	16	25	11	17	11	6	17	12
C66	Malignant neoplasm of ureter	M	166	16	35	25	13	19	15	13	21	9
		F	92	11	21	14	6	10	5	5	5	15
C67	Malignant neoplasm of bladder	M	6,317	328	1,069	710	564	538	718	626	1,021	743
		F	2,515	162	424	275	231	227	249	245	393	309
C68	Malignant neoplasm of other and unspecified urinery organs	M	83	3	18	3	10	6	9	8	10	16
		F	28	1	2	1	4	3	5	3	6	3
C69	Malignant neoplasm of eye and adnexa	M	186	4	20	20	21	19	12	22	28	40
		F	158	6	16	7	13	16	14	22	22	42
C70	Malignant neoplasm of meninges	M	25	1	5	1	3	2	4	3	2	4
		F	49	-	11	5	3	1	12	7	7	3
C71	Malignant neoplasm of brain	M	2,032	122	270	229	166	190	216	245	353	241
		F	1,505	86	225	162	128	122	170	189	261	162
C72	Malignant neoplasm of spinal cord, cranial nerves and other parts of central nervous system	M	55	2	2	8	4	5	9	8	9	8
		F	52	2	4	4	10	7	7	7	8	3
C73	Malignant neoplasm of thyroid gland	M	316	13	41	33	21	39	34	45	53	37
		F	862	42	125	106	66	98	96	129	134	66
C74	Malignant neoplasm of adrenal gland	M	79	7	8	5	6	5	9	7	17	15
		F	98	7	15	6	10	8	9	12	18	13
C75	Malignant neoplasm of other endocrine glands and related structures	M	39	2	6	7	3	2	3	1	6	9
		F	34	1	2	5	1	4	3	3	8	7

Table 4 Registrations in government offices for the regions - *continued*

ICD (10th Revision) number	Site description		England	North East	North West	Yorkshire and the Humber	East Midlands	West Midlands	East of England	London	South East	South West
C76	Malignant neoplasm of other and ill-defined sites	M F	207 327	4 6	19 30	6 13	13 15	5 18	24 46	60 95	44 62	32 42
C77	Secondary and unspecified malignant neoplasm of lymph nodes	M F	363 285	33 17	58 44	43 27	36 28	34 31	26 34	37 18	47 44	49 42
C78	Secondary malignant neoplasm of respiratory and digestive organs	M F	1,901 2,186	139 176	253 203	205 272	257 257	167 193	259 244	184 224	314 365	123 252
C79	Secondary malignant neoplasm of other sites	M F	891 884	63 60	57 63	103 108	86 85	66 99	95 101	112 110	180 156	129 102
C80	Malignant neoplasm without specification of site	M F	2,300 3,040	91 149	473 571	216 299	122 193	275 369	235 335	249 340	328 432	311 352
C81	Hodgkin's disease	M F	669 507	32 25	87 67	75 48	56 38	61 43	74 56	104 72	111 90	69 68
C82-C85	Non-Hodgkin's lymphoma	M F	4,146 3,648	196 195	493 436	426 345	353 336	398 351	431 387	505 442	740 662	604 494
C82	Follicular (nodular) non-Hodgkin's lymphoma	M F	524 558	19 35	69 57	58 62	45 52	52 57	47 50	47 51	108 104	79 90
C83	Diffuse non-Hodgkin's lymphoma	M F	1,487 1,196	98 77	151 134	185 139	155 130	170 146	112 85	123 100	285 244	208 141
C84	Peripheral and cutaneous T-cell lymphomas	M F	273 176	7 12	25 19	29 25	32 21	41 27	37 9	23 17	35 22	44 24
C85	Other and unspecified types on non-Hodgkin's lymphoma	M F	1,862 1,718	72 71	248 226	154 119	121 133	135 121	235 243	312 274	312 292	273 239
C88	Malignant immunoproliferative diseases	M F	133 74	4 1	9 2	9 8	8 8	9 5	8 5	20 8	37 25	29 12
C90	Multiple myeloma and malignant plasma cell neoplasms	M F	1,528 1,331	74 61	165 157	174 157	128 116	146 130	164 124	187 165	276 238	214 183
C91-C95	All leukaemias	M F	3,159 2,439	135 130	340 279	378 306	253 181	338 240	315 231	380 287	645 487	375 298
C91	Lymphoid leukaemia	M F	1,632 1,163	64 58	156 103	222 170	143 67	170 121	150 103	170 131	345 249	212 161
C92	Myeloid leukaemia	M F	1,368 1,137	66 61	164 159	150 127	102 106	145 99	150 118	187 138	262 209	142 120
C93	Monocytic leukaemia	M F	42 39	- 1	- -	2 5	2 2	7 7	3 2	12 8	13 9	3 5
C94	Other leukaemias of specified cell type	M F	21 11	1 2	4 1	1 -	1 -	4 3	1 -	5 1	3 4	1 -
C95	Leukaemia of unspecified cell type	M F	96 89	4 8	16 16	3 4	5 6	12 10	11 8	6 9	22 16	17 12
C96	Other and unspecified malignant neoplasms of lymphoid, haematopoietic and related tissue	M F	19 15	- -	- -	2 -	1 2	2 2	3 2	7 4	2 3	2 2
C97	Malignant neoplasms of independent (primary) multiple sites	M F	- -	- -	- -	- -	- -	- -	- -	- -	- -	- -
D00	Carcinoma in situ of oral cavity, oesophagus and stomach	M F	109 88	8 5	16 12	13 12	10 5	13 4	6 12	10 9	12 10	21 19
D01	Carcinoma in situ of other and unspecified digestive organs	M F	195 180	9 9	20 23	11 6	9 9	28 29	22 19	30 18	46 41	20 26
D02	Carcinoma in situ of middle ear and respiratory system	M F	163 49	5 1	35 17	25 8	14 4	15 1	7 1	14 3	15 7	33 7
D03	Melanoma in situ	M F	760 1,112	45 54	88 138	66 109	96 126	63 102	86 98	34 51	131 200	151 234

Table 4 Registrations in government offices for the regions - *continued*

ICD (10th Revision) number	Site description		England	North East	North West	Yorkshire and the Humber	East Midlands	West Midlands	East of England	London	South East	South West
D04	Carcinoma in situ of skin	M F	**1,890** **3,741**	127 305	453 955	273 610	245 392	238 499	227 423	111 155	216 402	- -
D05	Carcinoma in situ of breast	M F	**17** **3,019**	5 127	3 363	3 332	4 268	- 271	- 342	- 354	2 508	- 454
D06	Carcinoma in situ of cervix uteri	F	**19,517**	1,527	2,830	2,052	1,868	2,580	1,892	2,073	2,672	2,023
D07	Carcinoma in situ of other and unspecified genital organs	M F	**406** **611**	35 32	36 118	45 57	27 60	65 68	41 53	42 50	62 80	53 93
D09	Carcinoma in situ of other and unspecified sites	M F	**2,243** **787**	320 104	455 167	433 167	54 13	70 20	169 62	284 107	338 111	120 36
D33	Benign neoplasm of brain and other parts of central nervous system	M F	**235** **249**	18 12	18 17	20 18	22 23	16 17	27 41	19 25	54 50	41 46
D35.2	Benign neoplasm of pituitary gland	M F	**201** **156**	8 11	29 21	28 26	28 23	25 17	19 11	27 25	37 22	- -
D35.3	Benign neoplasm of cranio-pharyngeal duct	M F	- -	- -	- -	- -	- -	- -	- -	- -	- -	- -
D35.4	Benign neoplasm of pineal gland	M F	- -	- -	- -	- -	- -	- -	- -	- -	- -	- -
D37	Neoplasm of uncertain or unknown behaviour of oral cavity and digestive organs	M F	**654** **691**	21 39	222 171	42 42	57 74	41 42	38 36	32 37	99 142	102 108
D38	Neoplasm of uncertain or unknown behaviour of middle ear and respiratory and intrathoracic organs	M F	**71** **68**	- -	16 9	4 2	1 6	3 3	2 3	- 3	20 21	25 21
D39	Neoplasm of uncertain or unknown behaviour of female genital organs	F	**303**	9	55	11	31	24	40	21	45	67
D40	Neoplasm of uncertain or unknown behaviour of male genital organs	M	**93**	3	21	4	3	2	6	17	15	22
D41	Neoplasm of uncertain or unknown behaviour of urinary organs	M F	**1,859** **746**	- -	28 12	96 44	288 123	448 183	277 92	6 2	292 112	424 178
D42	Neoplasm of uncertain or unknown behaviour of meninges	M F	**18** **23**	1 -	3 3	- -	2 1	9 9	- 2	1 2	1 1	1 5
D43	Neoplasm of uncertain or unknown behaviour of brain and central nervous system	M F	**259** **249**	13 6	43 42	19 20	20 16	27 39	14 19	26 21	50 43	47 43
D44	Neoplasm of uncertain or unknown behaviour of endocrine glands	M F	**90** **103**	2 5	13 12	8 8	5 9	8 7	4 8	3 4	18 21	29 29
D45	Polycythaemia vera	M F	**199** **156**	3 11	16 17	16 14	28 15	27 15	15 13	20 28	63 38	11 5
D46	Myelodysplastic syndromes	M F	**1,104** **1,005**	45 34	105 115	128 111	110 117	81 61	110 85	111 84	191 167	223 231
D47	Other neoplasms of uncertain or unknown behaviour of lymphoid, haematopoietic and related tissue	M F	**872** **1,009**	31 31	51 54	170 208	49 54	40 64	82 87	107 140	215 236	127 135
D48	Neoplasm of uncertain or unknown behaviour of other and unspecified sites	M F	**243** **367**	3 5	18 54	12 9	36 32	9 18	6 18	14 30	63 87	82 114
O01	Hydatidiform mole	F	**241**	15	32	27	19	-	1	57	31	59

Table 5 Rates per 100,000 population of newly diagnosed cases of cancer: site, sex and government office for the region of residence, 2001

England, government offices for the regions Registered by May 2004

ICD (10th Revision) number	Site description		England	North East	North West	Yorkshire and the Humber	East Midlands	West Midlands	East of England	London	South East	South West
	All registrations	M	625.7	746.2	684.2	685.3	637.0	638.8	579.2	396.3	607.8	824.8
		F	673.9	802.3	738.9	734.3	701.3	691.5	621.5	443.4	645.7	855.9
C00-C97	All cancers	M	577.3	688.7	632.8	626.7	583.2	591.3	535.5	371.1	558.4	761.0
		F	537.3	621.7	588.6	581.9	546.6	540.2	499.5	354.5	522.6	700.8
C00-C97 xC44	All cancers excluding nmsc	M	466.0	548.3	497.7	492.7	453.3	462.0	446.0	355.9	466.2	556.0
		F	444.2	496.2	464.8	467.6	444.7	430.3	431.7	345.0	448.6	531.5
C00-C14	Malignant neoplasm of lip, mouth and pharynx	M	10.8	13.4	13.7	11.4	10.2	10.6	9.2	9.0	10.3	10.8
		F	5.8	5.6	6.6	6.6	5.9	6.0	4.7	5.2	5.4	6.3
C00	Malignant neoplasm of lip	M	0.7	1.2	0.6	1.2	0.6	0.6	0.8	0.1	0.7	0.6
		F	0.3	0.9	0.2	0.6	0.1	0.1	0.4	0.2	0.4	0.2
C01	Malignant neoplasm of base of tongue	M	0.8	1.1	0.9	0.9	1.1	0.7	0.7	0.6	0.5	0.7
		F	0.2	0.2	0.3	0.3	0.1	0.3	0.3	0.2	0.2	0.2
C02	Malignant neoplasm of other and unspecified parts of tongue	M	1.8	2.1	2.2	1.9	1.7	1.6	1.4	1.6	1.9	2.2
		F	1.2	0.4	1.1	1.4	1.2	1.4	1.1	1.2	1.2	1.2
C03	Malignant neoplasm of gum	M	0.4	0.1	0.3	0.2	0.6	0.3	0.8	0.5	0.5	0.3
		F	0.3	0.2	0.3	0.3	0.6	0.4	0.3	0.3	0.3	0.4
C04	Malignant neoplasm of floor of mouth	M	1.0	1.8	1.8	1.0	0.8	1.0	0.6	0.7	0.9	0.6
		F	0.4	0.4	0.6	0.4	0.6	0.4	0.3	0.4	0.3	0.5
C05	Malignant neoplasm of palate	M	0.5	0.7	0.8	0.3	0.5	0.5	0.3	0.4	0.4	0.7
		F	0.4	0.8	0.4	0.5	0.5	0.2	0.3	0.2	0.4	0.6
C06	Malignant neoplasm of other and unspecified parts of mouth	M	0.8	0.7	1.3	1.3	0.7	0.5	0.6	0.8	0.7	0.8
		F	0.6	0.5	0.8	0.6	0.8	0.5	0.3	0.6	0.7	0.5
C07	Malignant neoplasm of parotid gland	M	0.8	0.7	0.6	1.0	0.6	0.8	0.7	0.7	1.2	0.9
		F	0.6	0.8	0.5	0.9	0.6	0.6	0.4	0.6	0.3	0.7
C08	Malignant neoplasm of other and unspecified major salivary glands	M	0.2	0.2	0.2	0.2	0.3	0.2	0.1	0.2	0.3	0.3
		F	0.2	0.2	0.2	0.1	0.3	0.3	0.1	0.2	0.2	0.3
C09	Malignant neoplasm of tonsil	M	1.4	1.9	1.8	1.1	0.7	1.5	1.5	1.2	1.2	1.5
		F	0.5	0.5	0.5	0.5	0.2	0.7	0.3	0.3	0.4	0.6
C10	Malignant neoplasm of oropharynx	M	0.4	0.7	0.6	0.4	0.7	0.7	0.2	0.3	0.3	0.2
		F	0.1	0.1	0.1	0.1	0.1	0.1	0.1	0.1	0.1	0.1
C11	Malignant neoplasm of nasopharynx	M	0.4	0.3	0.3	0.2	0.6	0.5	0.5	0.4	0.3	0.9
		F	0.3	-	0.4	0.2	0.1	0.3	0.1	0.3	0.2	0.4
C12	Malignant neoplasm of piriform sinus	M	0.7	1.1	0.9	0.8	0.5	1.1	0.6	0.5	0.6	0.3
		F	0.1	0.2	0.2	0.1	0.1	0.2	0.1	0.1	0.1	0.1
C13	Malignant neoplasm of hypopharynx	M	0.3	0.6	0.5	0.5	0.2	0.4	0.1	0.3	0.3	0.2
		F	0.3	0.4	0.4	0.4	0.3	0.1	0.3	0.2	0.2	0.3
C14	Malignant neoplasm of other and ill-defined sites in the lip, oral cavity and pharynx	M	0.5	0.3	0.8	0.3	0.6	0.3	0.2	0.6	0.4	0.5
		F	0.2	-	0.3	0.4	0.1	0.1	0.1	0.3	0.3	0.2
C15	Malignant neoplasm of oesophagus	M	15.8	13.6	19.1	15.1	18.3	16.1	13.5	10.6	16.2	19.9
		F	9.0	9.6	10.5	8.8	9.7	9.7	7.5	6.5	9.2	10.5
C16	Malignant neoplasm of stomach	M	19.6	26.4	24.1	21.4	20.9	22.1	18.7	15.4	15.4	18.8
		F	10.4	16.4	12.3	13.2	10.6	10.7	9.0	8.0	8.2	9.8
C17	Malignant neoplasm of small intestine	M	1.3	1.5	1.4	1.4	0.8	1.7	1.1	0.9	1.3	1.8
		F	1.1	0.8	1.2	1.2	1.1	1.0	1.1	0.7	1.1	1.7
C18-C20	Malignant neoplasm of colon and rectum	M	61.4	79.6	68.4	65.5	60.8	66.6	58.9	43.2	56.8	71.5
		F	50.3	56.6	51.1	52.5	47.9	47.4	51.3	36.1	52.7	64.4
C18	Malignant neoplasm of colon	M	36.7	44.0	40.6	36.7	35.3	39.0	33.7	26.3	34.6	48.6
		F	34.4	37.1	35.1	33.4	33.0	32.4	33.3	24.2	36.8	48.2
C19	Malignant neoplasm of rectosigmoid junction	M	5.0	8.8	5.9	6.7	5.2	3.9	5.3	3.7	4.7	3.2
		F	3.4	4.9	3.3	4.9	2.9	2.7	4.3	2.9	2.9	2.4

Table 5 Registrations in government offices for the regions - *continued*

ICD (10th Revision) number	Site description		England	North East	North West	Yorkshire and the Humber	East Midlands	West Midlands	East of England	London	South East	South West
C20	Malignant neoplasm of rectum	M F	**19.8** **12.6**	26.8 14.6	21.8 12.7	22.1 14.3	20.3 12.0	23.7 12.2	20.0 13.7	13.2 9.0	17.5 12.9	19.7 13.8
C21	Malignant neoplasm of anus and anal canal	M F	**1.1** **1.5**	1.5 1.6	1.0 1.7	1.3 1.1	1.0 1.2	0.7 1.5	0.5 0.9	1.5 1.4	1.0 1.8	1.1 2.4
C22	Malignant neoplasm of liver and intrahepatic bile ducts	M F	**5.1** **3.5**	6.5 4.7	6.9 6.5	5.0 2.9	4.5 3.6	4.5 3.0	3.5 2.3	5.5 3.2	4.7 2.3	5.6 3.3
C23	Malignant neoplasm of gallbladder	M F	**0.5** **1.1**	1.1 1.0	0.2 1.2	0.7 1.7	0.7 1.0	0.5 1.0	0.5 0.9	0.4 0.9	0.5 1.3	0.4 1.1
C24	Malignant neoplasm of other and unspecified parts of biliary tract	M F	**1.2** **1.2**	1.4 1.3	1.0 0.7	0.9 1.2	1.1 0.8	1.0 1.1	1.1 1.3	1.1 1.0	1.6 1.5	1.7 2.1
C25	Malignant neoplasm of pancreas	M F	**11.6** **11.8**	13.3 13.2	11.2 10.9	12.0 13.5	13.4 11.9	10.8 11.0	10.4 12.9	9.7 10.4	11.5 11.8	14.9 12.7
C26	Malignant neoplasm of other and ill-defined digestive organs	M F	**1.0** **1.3**	0.2 0.2	1.1 1.1	0.6 0.5	1.1 0.9	0.4 0.6	0.4 1.2	1.0 1.4	1.4 2.1	1.7 2.7
C30	Malignant neoplasm of nasal cavity and middle ear	M F	**0.4** **0.3**	0.7 0.5	0.4 0.4	0.3 0.3	0.2 0.1	0.2 0.3	0.6 0.3	0.3 0.2	0.6 0.6	0.4 0.5
C31	Malignant neoplasm of accessory sinuses	M F	**0.4** **0.2**	0.3 0.2	0.4 0.3	0.4 -	0.3 0.1	0.3 0.3	0.3 0.1	0.3 0.2	0.4 0.2	0.5 0.3
C32	Malignant neoplasm of larynx	M F	**6.1** **1.3**	9.6 2.0	7.9 1.8	7.4 1.5	5.8 1.4	6.7 1.0	5.2 1.2	4.5 1.3	5.3 1.0	5.2 0.9
C33-C34	Malignant neoplasm of trachea, bronchus and lung	M F	**76.9** **47.4**	113.0 75.2	90.9 61.1	88.4 57.8	76.0 45.7	76.1 42.1	67.0 40.3	63.8 38.8	67.6 40.1	75.7 42.8
C33	Malignant neoplasm of trachea	M F	**0.1** **0.1**	0.1 0.1	0.3 0.3	0.1 0.1	0.2 0.0	0.2 0.0	0.1 0.1	0.0 0.1	0.2 0.0	0.0 0.1
C34	Malignant neoplasm of bronchus and lung	M F	**76.8** **47.3**	112.9 75.2	90.5 60.9	88.3 57.7	75.8 45.7	76.0 42.1	66.9 40.2	63.8 38.7	67.4 40.1	75.6 42.7
C37	Malignant neoplasm of thymus	M F	**0.1** **0.1**	0.2 0.2	0.0 0.1	0.3 0.1	0.2 0.1	0.1 0.2	0.1 0.1	0.1 0.1	0.1 0.0	0.2 0.2
C38	Malignant neoplasm of heart, mediastinum and pleura	M F	**0.6** **0.4**	0.5 0.1	0.9 0.7	0.5 0.4	0.4 0.3	0.4 0.1	0.3 0.2	0.2 0.3	0.6 0.4	1.3 0.7
C39	Malignant neoplasm of other and ill-defined sites in the respiratory system and intrathoracic organs	M F	**0.0** **0.0**	- -	- 0.0	- -	- -	- 0.0	- 0.0	0.1 -	- -	0.0 -
C40	Malignant neoplasm of bone and articular cartilage of limbs	M F	**0.5** **0.4**	0.7 0.5	0.5 0.2	0.3 0.4	0.5 0.2	0.6 0.5	0.4 0.2	0.5 0.4	0.4 0.3	0.5 0.6
C41	Malignant neoplasm of bone and articular cartilage of other and unspecified sites	M F	**0.5** **0.5**	0.5 0.2	0.8 1.0	0.3 0.2	0.4 0.5	0.2 0.4	0.6 0.4	0.3 0.2	0.4 0.4	0.7 0.6
C43	Malignant melanoma of skin	M F	**10.9** **13.6**	8.6 14.5	8.6 12.2	10.6 14.0	9.2 12.3	10.8 11.9	10.8 13.5	6.4 7.5	13.7 15.8	19.6 22.8
C44	Other malignant neoplasms of skin	M F	**111.3** **93.2**	140.5 125.6	135.1 123.8	134.0 114.3	129.9 101.9	129.3 109.9	89.5 67.8	15.1 9.5	92.2 74.0	205.0 169.2
C45	Mesothelioma	M F	**5.9** **1.3**	9.5 1.7	6.8 1.1	6.0 1.3	4.6 1.2	4.6 1.0	6.3 1.5	3.8 1.2	6.8 1.7	6.5 1.3
C46	Kaposi's sarcoma	M F	**0.3** **0.1**	0.1 -	0.1 0.1	0.0 -	0.1 -	0.3 -	0.2 0.0	0.9 0.4	0.2 -	0.1 -
C47	Malignant neoplasm of peripheral nerves and autonomic nervous system	M F	**0.2** **0.2**	0.3 0.3	0.1 0.1	0.2 0.2	0.3 0.2	0.2 0.2	0.1 0.1	0.1 0.1	0.1 0.2	0.3 0.2
C48	Malignant neoplasm of retroperitoneum and peritoneum	M F	**0.4** **0.7**	0.2 1.5	0.5 0.7	0.3 0.6	0.3 1.1	0.4 0.7	0.3 0.7	0.3 0.6	0.5 0.5	0.5 0.7

Table 5 Registrations in government offices for the regions - *continued*

ICD (10th Revision) number	Site description		England	North East	North West	Yorkshire and the Humber	East Midlands	West Midlands	East of England	London	South East	South West
C49	Malignant neoplasm of other connective and soft tissue	M F	**2.2** **1.9**	2.1 1.2	2.3 1.6	2.6 2.1	2.4 2.1	2.0 2.0	1.9 1.9	1.1 1.1	2.0 1.8	4.2 3.2
C50	Malignant neoplasm of breast	M F	**1.0** **136.1**	1.3 132.2	0.9 137.6	0.6 131.0	0.3 135.3	1.3 137.0	1.1 137.8	1.0 108.1	1.1 144.2	1.4 166.5
C51	Malignant neoplasm of vulva	F	**3.4**	5.2	3.8	3.3	4.1	3.9	3.0	1.8	3.1	4.5
C52	Malignant neoplasm of vagina	F	**0.7**	0.9	0.9	0.7	0.8	0.7	0.5	0.4	0.7	0.6
C53	Malignant neoplasm of cervix uteri	F	**9.6**	11.7	11.6	11.9	10.3	11.4	7.0	7.4	7.1	11.0
C54	Malignant neoplasm of corpus uteri	F	**18.5**	15.3	18.0	17.2	22.4	19.6	20.8	13.7	17.4	24.5
C55	Malignant neoplasm of uterus, part unspecified	F	**1.1**	1.5	1.4	1.7	1.1	1.2	0.9	0.7	0.9	0.7
C56-C57	Malignant neoplasm of ovary and other unspecified female genital organs	F	**22.7**	23.9	21.2	24.7	23.0	23.7	23.1	16.2	24.8	26.8
C56	Malignant neoplasm of ovary	F	**22.3**	23.7	20.9	24.5	22.7	23.2	22.8	15.8	24.3	26.0
C57	Malignant neoplasm of other and unspecified female genital organs	F	**0.4**	0.2	0.3	0.2	0.3	0.5	0.3	0.4	0.5	0.8
C58	Malignant neoplasm of placenta	F	**0.0**	-	0.0	-	-	0.0	0.1	0.0	0.0	-
C60	Malignant neoplasm of penis	M	**1.4**	1.7	1.4	2.0	1.6	1.4	1.5	0.7	1.1	1.7
C61	Malignant neoplasm of prostate	M	**107.8**	113.1	105.4	104.8	94.2	113.4	114.3	80.5	115.6	138.0
C62	Malignant neoplasm of testis	M	**6.8**	7.4	5.9	7.5	6.5	6.1	6.1	6.1	7.7	8.8
C63	Malignant neoplasm of other and unspecified male genital organs	M	**0.2**	0.2	0.3	0.2	0.4	0.4	0.3	0.1	0.1	0.2
C64	Malignant neoplasm of kidney, except renal pelvis	M F	**11.2** **6.5**	13.8 8.2	10.4 7.0	12.3 9.0	12.6 5.6	10.7 5.1	9.7 6.8	7.8 5.2	12.2 6.1	14.2 7.3
C65	Malignant neoplasm of renal pelvis	M F	**0.8** **0.5**	2.0 0.5	0.8 0.5	1.6 1.0	0.9 0.5	0.7 0.6	0.6 0.4	0.4 0.2	0.9 0.4	0.5 0.5
C66	Malignant neoplasm of ureter	M F	**0.7** **0.4**	1.3 0.8	1.1 0.6	1.0 0.5	0.6 0.3	0.7 0.4	0.6 0.2	0.4 0.1	0.5 0.1	0.4 0.6
C67	Malignant neoplasm of bladder	M F	**26.2** **10.0**	26.8 12.5	32.5 12.2	29.4 10.8	27.4 10.9	20.8 8.4	27.1 9.0	17.4 6.6	26.0 9.6	30.9 12.2
C68	Malignant neoplasm of other and unspecified urinery organs	M F	**0.3** **0.1**	0.2 0.1	0.5 0.1	0.1 0.1	0.5 0.0	0.2 0.2	0.3 0.2	0.2 0.1	0.3 0.1	0.7 0.1
C69	Malignant neoplasm of eye and adnexa	M F	**0.8** **0.6**	0.3 0.5	0.6 0.5	0.8 0.3	1.0 0.6	0.7 0.6	0.5 0.5	0.6 0.6	0.7 0.5	1.7 1.7
C70	Malignant neoplasm of meninges	M F	**0.1** **0.2**	0.1 -	0.2 0.3	0.0 0.2	0.1 0.1	0.1 0.0	0.2 0.4	0.1 0.2	0.1 0.2	0.2 0.1
C71	Malignant neoplasm of brain	M F	**8.4** **6.0**	10.0 6.6	8.2 6.5	9.5 6.3	8.1 6.0	7.3 4.5	8.2 6.2	6.8 5.1	9.0 6.4	10.0 6.4
C72	Malignant neoplasm of spinal cord, cranial nerves and other parts of central nervous system	M F	**0.2** **0.2**	0.2 0.2	0.1 0.1	0.3 0.2	0.2 0.5	0.2 0.3	0.3 0.3	0.2 0.2	0.2 0.2	0.3 0.1
C73	Malignant neoplasm of thyroid gland	M F	**1.3** **3.4**	1.1 3.2	1.2 3.6	1.4 4.2	1.0 3.1	1.5 3.6	1.3 3.5	1.3 3.5	1.4 3.3	1.5 2.6
C74	Malignant neoplasm of adrenal gland	M F	**0.3** **0.4**	0.6 0.5	0.2 0.4	0.2 0.2	0.3 0.5	0.2 0.3	0.3 0.3	0.2 0.3	0.4 0.4	0.6 0.5
C75	Malignant neoplasm of other endocrine glands and related structures	M F	**0.2** **0.1**	0.2 0.1	0.2 0.1	0.3 0.2	0.1 0.0	0.1 0.1	0.1 0.1	0.0 0.1	0.2 0.2	0.4 0.3

Table 5 Registrations in government offices for the regions - *continued*

ICD (10th Revision) number	Site description		England	North East	North West	Yorkshire and the Humber	East Midlands	West Midlands	East of England	London	South East	South West
C76	Malignant neoplasm of other and ill-defined sites	M F	**0.9** **1.3**	0.3 0.5	0.6 0.9	0.2 0.5	0.6 0.7	0.2 0.7	0.9 1.7	1.7 2.6	1.1 1.5	1.3 1.7
C77	Secondary and unspecified malignant neoplasm of lymph nodes	M F	**1.5** **1.1**	2.7 1.3	1.8 1.3	1.8 1.1	1.7 1.3	1.3 1.2	1.0 1.2	1.0 0.5	1.2 1.1	2.0 1.7
C78	Secondary malignant neoplasm of respiratory and digestive organs	M F	**7.9** **8.7**	11.4 13.6	7.7 5.8	8.5 10.7	12.5 12.1	6.4 7.2	9.8 8.9	5.1 6.0	8.0 8.9	5.1 9.9
C79	Secondary malignant neoplasm of other sites	M F	**3.7** **3.5**	5.2 4.6	1.7 1.8	4.3 4.2	4.2 4.0	2.5 3.7	3.6 3.7	3.1 3.0	4.6 3.8	5.4 4.0
C80	Malignant neoplasm without specification of site	M F	**9.5** **12.0**	7.4 11.5	14.4 16.4	8.9 11.7	5.9 9.1	10.6 13.7	8.9 12.2	6.9 9.2	8.4 10.5	12.9 13.9
C81	Hodgkin's disease	M F	**2.8** **2.0**	2.6 1.9	2.6 1.9	3.1 1.9	2.7 1.8	2.4 1.6	2.8 2.0	2.9 1.9	2.8 2.2	2.9 2.7
C82-C85	Non-Hodgkin's lymphoma	M F	**17.2** **14.4**	16.0 15.0	15.0 12.5	17.6 13.5	17.2 15.8	15.4 13.0	16.3 14.1	14.0 11.9	18.9 16.2	25.1 19.5
C82	Follicular (nodular) non-Hodgkin's lymphoma	M F	**2.2** **2.2**	1.6 2.7	2.1 1.6	2.4 2.4	2.2 2.4	2.0 2.1	1.8 1.8	1.3 1.4	2.8 2.5	3.3 3.6
C83	Diffuse non-Hodgkin's lymphoma lymphoma	M F	**6.2** **4.7**	8.0 5.9	4.6 3.8	7.7 5.4	7.5 6.1	6.6 5.4	4.2 3.1	3.4 2.7	7.3 6.0	8.7 5.6
C84	Peripheral and cutaneous T-cell lymphomas	M F	**1.1** **0.7**	0.6 0.9	0.8 0.5	1.2 1.0	1.6 1.0	1.6 1.0	1.4 0.3	0.6 0.5	0.9 0.5	1.8 0.9
C85	Other and unspecified types on non-Hodgkin's lymphoma	M F	**7.7** **6.8**	5.9 5.5	7.6 6.5	6.4 4.7	5.9 6.3	5.2 4.5	8.9 8.8	8.7 7.4	8.0 7.1	11.4 9.4
C88	Malignant immunoproliferative diseases	M F	**0.6** **0.3**	0.3 0.1	0.3 0.1	0.4 0.3	0.4 0.4	0.3 0.2	0.3 0.2	0.6 0.2	0.9 0.6	1.2 0.5
C90	Multiple myeloma and malignant plasma cell neoplasms	M F	**6.3** **5.3**	6.1 4.7	5.0 4.5	7.2 6.1	6.2 5.5	5.6 4.8	6.2 4.5	5.2 4.4	7.0 5.8	8.9 7.2
C91-C95	All leukaemias	M F	**13.1** **9.7**	11.1 10.0	10.4 8.0	15.6 12.0	12.3 8.5	13.0 8.9	11.9 8.4	10.6 7.7	16.4 11.9	15.6 11.8
C91	Lymphoid leukaemia	M F	**6.8** **4.6**	5.2 4.5	4.7 3.0	9.2 6.7	6.9 3.2	6.6 4.5	5.7 3.7	4.7 3.5	8.8 6.1	8.8 6.4
C92	Myeloid leukaemia	M F	**5.7** **4.5**	5.4 4.7	5.0 4.6	6.2 5.0	5.0 5.0	5.6 3.7	5.7 4.3	5.2 3.7	6.7 5.1	5.9 4.7
C93	Monocytic leukaemia	M F	**0.2** **0.2**	- 0.1	- -	0.1 0.2	0.1 0.1	0.3 0.3	0.1 0.1	0.3 0.2	0.3 0.2	0.1 0.2
C94	Other leukaemias of specified cell type	M F	**0.1** **0.0**	0.1 0.2	0.1 0.0	0.0 -	0.0 -	0.2 0.1	0.0 -	0.1 0.0	0.1 0.1	0.0 -
C95	Leukaemia of unspecified cell type	M F	**0.4** **0.4**	0.3 0.6	0.5 0.5	0.1 0.2	0.2 0.3	0.5 0.4	0.4 0.3	0.2 0.2	0.6 0.4	0.7 0.5
C96	Other and unspecified malignant neoplasms of lymphoid, haematopoietic and related tissue	M F	**0.1** **0.1**	- -	- -	0.1 -	0.0 0.1	0.1 0.1	0.1 0.1	0.2 0.1	0.1 0.1	0.1 0.1
C97	Malignant neoplasms of independent (primary) multiple sites	M F	**-** **-**	- -	- -	- -	- -	- -	- -	- -	- -	- -
D00	Carcinoma in situ of oral cavity, oesophagus and stomach	M F	**0.5** **0.3**	0.7 0.4	0.5 0.3	0.5 0.5	0.5 0.2	0.5 0.1	0.2 0.4	0.3 0.2	0.3 0.2	0.9 0.7
D01	Carcinoma in situ of other and unspecified digestive organs	M F	**0.8** **0.7**	0.7 0.7	0.6 0.7	0.5 0.2	0.4 0.4	1.1 1.1	0.8 0.7	0.8 0.5	1.2 1.0	0.8 1.0
D02	Carcinoma in situ of middle ear and respiratory system	M F	**0.7** **0.2**	0.4 0.1	1.1 0.5	1.0 0.3	0.7 0.2	0.6 0.0	0.3 0.0	0.4 0.1	0.4 0.2	1.4 0.3
D03	Melanoma in situ	M F	**3.1** **4.4**	3.7 4.2	2.7 4.0	2.7 4.3	4.7 5.9	2.4 3.8	3.2 3.6	0.9 1.4	3.3 4.9	6.3 9.2

Table 5 Registrations in government offices for the regions - *continued*

ICD (10th Revision) number	Site description		England	North East	North West	Yorkshire and the Humber	East Midlands	West Midlands	East of England	London	South East	South West
D04	Carcinoma in situ of skin	M	**7.8**	10.4	13.8	11.3	11.9	9.2	8.6	3.1	5.5	-
		F	**14.8**	23.5	27.4	23.9	18.4	18.5	15.4	4.2	9.8	-
D05	Carcinoma in situ of breast	M	**0.1**	0.4	0.1	0.1	0.2	-	-	-	0.1	-
		F	**12.0**	9.8	10.4	13.0	12.6	10.1	12.4	9.5	12.4	17.9
D06	Carcinoma in situ of cervix uteri	F	**77.3**	117.7	81.3	80.4	87.9	95.8	68.7	55.9	65.2	79.8
D07	Carcinoma in situ of other and unspecified genital organs	M	**1.7**	2.9	1.1	1.9	1.3	2.5	1.5	1.2	1.6	2.2
		F	**2.4**	2.5	3.4	2.2	2.8	2.5	1.9	1.3	2.0	3.7
D09	Carcinoma in situ of other and unspecified sites	M	**9.3**	26.2	13.9	17.9	2.6	2.7	6.4	7.9	8.6	5.0
		F	**3.1**	8.0	4.8	6.5	0.6	0.7	2.3	2.9	2.7	1.4
D33	Benign neoplasm of brain and other parts of central nervous system	M	**1.0**	1.5	0.5	0.8	1.1	0.6	1.0	0.5	1.4	1.7
		F	**1.0**	0.9	0.5	0.7	1.1	0.6	1.5	0.7	1.2	1.8
D35.2	Benign neoplasm of pituitary gland	M	**0.8**	0.7	0.9	1.2	1.4	1.0	0.7	0.8	0.9	-
		F	**0.6**	0.8	0.6	1.0	1.1	0.6	0.4	0.7	0.5	-
D35.3	Benign neoplasm of craniopharyngeal duct	M	**-**	-	-	-	-	-	-	-	-	-
		F	**-**	-	-	-	-	-	-	-	-	-
D35.4	Benign neoplasm of pineal gland	M	**-**	-	-	-	-	-	-	-	-	-
		F	**-**	-	-	-	-	-	-	-	-	-
D37	Neoplasm of uncertain or unknown behaviour of oral cavity and digestive organs	M	**2.7**	1.7	6.8	1.7	2.8	1.6	1.4	0.9	2.5	4.2
		F	**2.7**	3.0	4.9	1.6	3.5	1.6	1.3	1.0	3.5	4.3
D38	Neoplasm of uncertain or unknown behaviour of middle ear and respiratory and intrathoracic organs	M	**0.3**	-	0.5	0.2	0.0	0.1	0.1	-	0.5	1.0
		F	**0.3**	-	0.3	0.1	0.3	0.1	0.1	0.1	0.5	0.8
D39	Neoplasm of uncertain or unknown behaviour of female genital organs	F	**1.2**	0.7	1.6	0.4	1.5	0.9	1.5	0.6	1.1	2.6
D40	Neoplasm of uncertain or unknown behaviour of male genital organs	M	**0.4**	0.2	0.6	0.2	0.1	0.1	0.2	0.5	0.4	0.9
D41	Neoplasm of uncertain or unknown behaviour of urinary organs	M	**7.7**	-	0.9	4.0	14.0	17.3	10.5	0.2	7.4	17.6
		F	**3.0**	-	0.3	1.7	5.8	6.8	3.3	0.1	2.7	7.0
D42	Neoplasm of uncertain or unknown behaviour of meninges	M	**0.1**	0.1	0.1	-	0.1	0.3	-	0.0	0.0	0.0
		F	**0.1**	-	0.1	-	0.0	0.3	0.1	0.1	0.0	0.2
D43	Neoplasm of uncertain or unknown behaviour of brain and central nervous system	M	**1.1**	1.1	1.3	0.8	1.0	1.0	0.5	0.7	1.3	2.0
		F	**1.0**	0.5	1.2	0.8	0.8	1.4	0.7	0.6	1.0	1.7
D44	Neoplasm of uncertain or unknown behaviour of endocrine glands	M	**0.4**	0.2	0.4	0.3	0.2	0.3	0.2	0.1	0.5	1.2
		F	**0.4**	0.4	0.3	0.3	0.4	0.3	0.3	0.1	0.5	1.1
D45	Polycythaemia vera	M	**0.8**	0.2	0.5	0.7	1.4	1.0	0.6	0.6	1.6	0.5
		F	**0.6**	0.8	0.5	0.5	0.7	0.6	0.5	0.8	0.9	0.2
D46	Myelodysplastic syndromes	M	**4.6**	3.7	3.2	5.3	5.3	3.1	4.2	3.1	4.9	9.3
		F	**4.0**	2.6	3.3	4.3	5.5	2.3	3.1	2.3	4.1	9.1
D47	Other neoplasms of uncertain or unknown behaviour of lymphoid, haematopoietic and related tissue	M	**3.6**	2.5	1.6	7.0	2.4	1.5	3.1	3.0	5.5	5.3
		F	**4.0**	2.4	1.6	8.1	2.5	2.4	3.2	3.8	5.8	5.3
D48	Neoplasm of uncertain or unknown behaviour of other and unspecified sites	M	**1.0**	0.2	0.5	0.5	1.7	0.3	0.2	0.4	1.6	3.4
		F	**1.5**	0.4	1.6	0.4	1.5	0.7	0.7	0.8	2.1	4.5
O01	Hydatidiform mole	F	**1.0**	1.2	0.9	1.1	0.9	-	0.0	1.5	0.8	2.3

Table 6 Series MB1 no. 32

Table 6 Standardised registration ratios: site, sex and government office for the region of residence, 2001

England, government offices for the regions
Registered by May 2004

ICD (10th Revision) number	Site description	Sex	North East	North West	Yorkshire and the Humber	East Midlands	West Midlands	East of England	London	South East	South West
	All registrations	M	116	110	109	99	101	88	80	94	114
		F	117	109	108	104	103	91	75	93	115
C00-C97	All cancers	M	116	110	108	98	102	88	81	94	114
		F	113	109	107	101	100	91	80	94	115
C00-C97 xC44	All cancers excluding nmsc	M	114	107	105	95	98	91	97	97	103
		F	109	104	104	99	97	95	94	98	106
C00-C14	Malignant neoplasm of lip, mouth and pharynx	M	120	126	104	91	97	82	103	94	90
		F	95	113	113	101	103	80	107	91	97
C00	Malignant neoplasm of lip	M	181	97	175	86	87	110	26	109	77
		F	293	73	186	45	48	113	75	119	43
C01	Malignant neoplasm of base of tongue	M	134	118	112	135	94	90	105	65	84
		F	89	137	109	55	132	113	118	76	57
C02	Malignant neoplasm of other and unspecified parts of tongue	M	112	118	103	90	85	75	108	100	109
		F	32	96	114	101	121	92	118	101	89
C03	Malignant neoplasm of gum	M	18	76	47	129	79	182	146	107	68
		F	43	98	78	174	127	91	106	88	89
C04	Malignant neoplasm of floor of mouth	M	172	176	102	75	98	58	87	93	57
		F	89	142	83	132	97	76	102	79	101
C05	Malignant neoplasm of palate	M	129	159	66	105	92	51	92	86	128
		F	201	97	133	113	54	69	67	93	140
C06	Malignant neoplasm of other and unspecified parts of mouth	M	77	154	154	80	55	66	123	84	89
		F	77	135	99	127	82	54	124	107	76
C07	Malignant neoplasm of parotid gland	M	88	71	125	69	93	83	107	144	93
		F	132	85	156	106	110	75	113	58	113
C08	Malignant neoplasm of other and unspecified major salivary glands	M	69	93	90	146	101	48	102	121	116
		F	115	101	39	141	150	71	97	83	125
C09	Malignant neoplasm of tonsil	M	131	131	80	51	108	106	104	89	103
		F	112	116	100	50	159	61	84	93	124
C10	Malignant neoplasm of oropharynx	M	146	139	95	152	149	50	83	75	52
		F	65	124	101	121	64	123	111	83	94
C11	Malignant neoplasm of nasopharynx	M	71	68	55	128	103	116	118	68	183
		F	-	170	77	55	132	42	127	66	163
C12	Malignant neoplasm of piriform sinus	M	159	131	113	68	154	85	99	81	38
		F	157	139	54	97	129	74	114	83	75
C13	Malignant neoplasm of hypopharynx	M	171	159	139	58	130	34	98	92	45
		F	136	145	127	119	54	103	86	69	89
C14	Malignant neoplasm of other and ill-defined sites in the lip, oral cavity and pharynx	M	66	170	69	128	64	46	154	84	93
		F	-	118	160	58	31	58	166	137	86
C15	Malignant neoplasm of oesophagus	M	83	121	95	113	101	82	86	100	109
		F	105	116	97	107	108	81	91	98	99
C16	Malignant neoplasm of stomach	M	131	123	108	104	112	90	101	76	81
		F	155	118	126	102	103	84	97	76	81
C17	Malignant neoplasm of small intestine	M	109	107	103	61	125	83	91	97	122
		F	76	107	107	98	88	101	76	95	140
C18-C20	Malignant neoplasm of colon and rectum	M	126	111	106	96	107	91	90	90	100
		F	110	101	103	95	94	99	90	101	110
C18	Malignant neoplasm of colon	M	117	111	99	93	105	87	92	91	113
		F	106	101	96	96	94	94	89	103	121
C19	Malignant neoplasm of rectosigmoid junction	M	170	118	134	100	77	101	95	92	55
		F	143	98	144	86	82	125	109	84	61

50

Table 6 Standardised registration ratios - *continued*

ICD (10th Revision) number	Site description		North East	North West	Yorkshire and the Humber	East Midlands	West Midlands	East of England	London	South East	South West
C20	Malignant neoplasm of rectum	M F	131 114	110 101	111 112	100 95	119 97	96 106	86 90	86 99	86 95
C21	Malignant neoplasm of anus and anal canal	M F	135 103	98 110	124 71	94 76	69 97	48 60	176 109	89 113	90 142
C22	Malignant neoplasm of liver and intrahepatic bile ducts	M F	122 131	133 185	96 83	85 103	86 87	64 65	135 115	88 63	95 82
C23	Malignant neoplasm of gallbladder	M F	217 86	47 105	136 146	129 86	104 88	91 81	111 101	91 107	62 87
C24	Malignant neoplasm of other and unspecified parts of biliary tract	M F	113 106	84 61	72 99	86 66	86 92	86 105	119 100	127 119	117 145
C25	Malignant neoplasm of pancreas	M F	111 110	97 92	102 113	112 100	93 93	85 106	107 111	96 95	109 92
C26	Malignant neoplasm of other and ill-defined digestive organs	M F	26 12	120 87	65 42	115 73	45 44	41 87	134 133	138 152	147 174
C30	Malignant neoplasm of nasal cavity and middle ear	M F	174 129	88 114	79 78	57 40	56 74	140 81	98 56	138 163	80 131
C31	Malignant neoplasm of accessory sinuses	M F	85 72	114 161	110 -	76 44	82 157	78 66	110 133	107 99	119 115
C32	Malignant neoplasm of larynx	M F	150 149	127 133	119 113	92 103	107 79	81 87	94 128	84 75	75 62
C33-C34	Malignant neoplasm of trachea, bronchus and lung	M F	142 153	118 127	114 120	96 95	98 88	83 83	107 103	85 82	84 79
C33	Malignant neoplasm of trachea	M F	60 82	231 280	62 85	142 51	116 40	54 116	27 73	131 52	27 77
C34	Malignant neoplasm of bronchus and lung	M F	142 153	118 127	114 120	96 95	98 88	83 83	108 103	85 82	84 79
C37	Malignant neoplasm of thymus	M F	128 187	24 72	231 65	153 117	93 156	59 119	53 105	80 20	152 154
C38	Malignant neoplasm of heart, mediastinum and pleura	M F	86 20	158 171	95 111	76 73	68 38	45 55	41 104	106 92	202 171
C39	Malignant neoplasm of other and ill-defined sites in the respiratory system and intrathoracic organs	M F	- -	- 239	- -	- -	- 307	- 293	649 -	- -	212 -
C40	Malignant neoplasm of bone and articular cartilage of limbs	M F	140 129	111 64	71 109	114 53	124 135	81 61	106 105	82 95	97 170
C41	Malignant neoplasm of bone and articular cartilage of other and unspecified sites	M F	106 33	173 222	63 50	84 112	50 80	121 93	73 58	82 77	144 126
C43	Malignant melanoma of skin	M F	77 105	79 90	96 103	82 90	99 88	96 98	68 60	123 114	164 157
C44	Other malignant neoplasms of skin	M F	123 132	122 132	119 121	114 109	116 118	77 71	17 13	80 76	158 158
C45	Mesothelioma	M F	154 126	114 81	101<>98	76 93	76 76	101 111	84 111	113 123	95 84
C46	Kaposi's sarcoma	M F	32 -	48 86	16 -	37 -	120 -	58 53	328 570	78 -	48 -
C47	Malignant neoplasm of peripheral nerves and autonomic nervous system	M F	198 163	37 76	102 124	178 125	142 118	69 57	57 59	62 114	172 119
C48	Malignant neoplasm of retroperitoneum and peritoneum	M F	59 203	128 90	82 80	82 153	104 96	81 98	84 104	124 66	111 93

Table 6 Standardised registration ratios - *continued*

ICD (10th Revision) number	Site description		North East	North West	Yorkshire and the Humber	East Midlands	West Midlands	East of England	London	South East	South West
					Government office for the region						
C49	Malignant neoplasm of other connective and soft tissue	M F	94 66	104 88	119 113	105 111	92 110	84 98	59 64	86 94	169 156
C50	Malignant neoplasm of breast	M F	126 95	87 100	57 96	28 98	128 100	106 99	129 94	110 103	121 111
C51	Malignant neoplasm of vulva	F	148	111	96	120	114	85	63	85	116
C52	Malignant neoplasm of vagina	F	138	135	106	121	102	70	80	96	74
C53	Malignant neoplasm of cervix uteri	F	121	122	125	107	120	73	79	74	111
C54	Malignant neoplasm of corpus uteri	F	79	96	91	119	104	109	91	91	118
C55	Malignant neoplasm of uterus, part unspecified	F	140	131	156	103	106	78	79	81	60
C56-C57	Malignant neoplasm of ovary and other unspecified female genital organs	F	102	92	108	100	104	99	85	106	106
C56	Malignant neoplasm of ovary	F	103	93	109	100	103	100	85	106	105
C57	Malignant neoplasm of other and unspecified female genital organs	F	38	72	49	70	130	71	116	126	178
C58	Malignant neoplasm of placenta	F	-	126	-	-	163	319	89	107	-
C60	Malignant neoplasm of penis	M	121	99	143	110	103	105	65	78	107
C61	Malignant neoplasm of prostate	M	102	98	96	85	104	101	97	104	108
C62	Malignant neoplasm of testis	M	111	89	112	97	92	91	78	114	135
C63	Malignant neoplasm of other and unspecified male genital organs	M	106	122	73	169	171	113	78	33	81
C64	Malignant neoplasm of kidney, except renal pelvis	M F	119 122	93 107	109 136	109 85	95 77	83 101	88 97	106 90	112 98
C65	Malignant neoplasm of renal pelvis	M F	232 94	97 95	185 202	107 107	81 131	69 81	55 42	104 84	52 86
C66	Malignant neoplasm of ureter	M F	183 223	154 163	149 148	89 77	105 101	78 49	69 47	76 32	47 141
C67	Malignant neoplasm of bladder	M F	100 124	125 122	111 107	102 109	79 85	98 88	86 84	96 92	100 104
C68	Malignant neoplasm of other and unspecified urinery organs	M F	70 71	160 52	36 35	137 171	67 102	94 159	83 88	72 125	164 92
C69	Malignant neoplasm of eye and adnexa	M F	41 72	78 73	106 43	130 97	94 94	57 79	94 112	91 84	197 240
C70	Malignant neoplasm of meninges	M F	78 -	147 162	40 100	139 72	74 19	142 219	91 118	48 85	147 54
C71	Malignant neoplasm of brain	M F	115 108	97 107	112 105	94 100	86 75	94 102	93 98	106 105	110 99
C72	Malignant neoplasm of spinal cord, cranial nerves and other parts of central nervous system	M F	72 74	27 55	145 75	85 227	84 125	148 122	102 98	100 94	143 56
C73	Malignant neoplasm of thyroid gland	M F	80 94	96 106	104 122	77 91	115 108	96 101	106 105	102 95	109 74
C74	Malignant neoplasm of adrenal gland	M F	173 137	74 110	63 60	88 120	58 76	101 83	67 91	131 112	179 127
C75	Malignant neoplasm of other endocrine glands and related structures	M F	99 56	113 42	178 144	89 35	48 110	69 80	18 65	95 144	222 197

Table 6 Standardised registration ratios - *continued*

ICD (10th Revision) number	Site description		North East	North West	Yorkshire and the Humber	East Midlands	West Midlands	East of England	London	South East	South West
C76	Malignant neoplasm of other and ill-defined sites	M F	38 36	69 67	29 39	73 55	23 52	101 126	231 241	126 111	135 111
C77	Secondary and unspecified malignant neoplasm of lymph nodes	M F	173 113	117 111	117 93	113 115	86 102	63 107	85 52	78 92	120 130
C78	Secondary malignant neoplasm of respiratory and digestive organs	M F	141 154	99 67	107 122	154 139	81 83	118 100	84 88	98 98	55 99
C79	Secondary malignant neoplasm of other sites	M F	136 128	47 51	115 119	110 113	69 104	92 102	108 106	120 105	124 100
C80	Malignant neoplasm without specification of site	M F	77 95	153 136	93 96	61 76	111 115	88 98	93 96	84 83	114 98
C81	Hodgkin's disease	M F	95 96	97 96	113 94	98 90	86 80	101 103	101 93	102 110	104 135
C82-C85	Non-Hodgkin's lymphoma	M F	91 101	87 86	102 93	97 108	89 90	91 95	100 99	107 109	130 120
C82	Follicular (nodular) non-Hodgkin's lymphoma	M F	69 118	96 73	109 109	98 109	91 95	79 80	72 74	124 112	139 147
C83	Diffuse non-Hodgkin's lymphoma	M F	126 122	74 80	123 114	119 128	106 114	66 64	67 69	115 122	125 104
C84	Peripheral and cutaneous T-cell lymphomas	M F	50 130	67 78	105 140	134 141	139 144	119 46	68 75	77 75	145 125
C85	Other and unspecified types on non-Hodgkin's lymphoma	M F	74 79	98 95	82 68	74 91	67 66	110 127	138 132	100 101	129 122
C88	Malignant immunoproliferative diseases	M F	59 26	50 20	67 106	69 128	63 63	52 60	131 93	164 198	183 137
C90	Multiple myeloma and malignant plasma cell neoplasms	M F	93 87	79 85	113 115	95 103	88 91	93 83	106 106	108 106	121 118
C91-C95	All leukaemias	M F	83 103	79 83	119 123	92 88	99 92	87 85	98 95	122 119	105 108
C91	Lymphoid leukaemia	M F	76 97	70 64	135 143	101 68	96 97	80 79	85 91	127 127	115 122
C92	Myeloid leukaemia	M F	94 103	89 101	109 110	86 110	99 82	96 93	109 98	115 109	92 93
C93	Monocytic leukaemia	M F	- 50	- -	47 127	55 61	154 171	63 46	226 160	187 136	65 113
C94	Other leukaemias of specified cell type	M F	91 342	140 65	47 -	55 -	176 256	42<>-	185 78	87 216	44 -
C95	Leukaemia of unspecified cell type	M F	83 177	126 131	31 44	60 81	117 106	99 80	52 86	135 104	150 113
C96	Other and unspecified malignant neoplasms of lymphoid, haematopoietic and related tissue	M F	- -	- -	105 -	61 158	98 124	139 120	280 211	63 120	95 120
C97	Malignant neoplasms of independent (primary) multiple sites	M F	- -	- -	- -	- -	- -	- -	- -	- -	- -
D00	Carcinoma in situ of oral cavity, oesophagus and stomach	M F	139 109	107 98	117 133	104 67	109 43	48 122	80 87	66 67	168 185
D01	Carcinoma in situ of other and unspecified digestive organs	M F	89 95	75 92	56 33	53 59	132 150	98 94	129 83	142 136	90 127
D02	Carcinoma in situ of middle ear and respiratory system	M F	58 38	156 247	151 159	97 95	84 19	37 18	74 52	56 86	178 126
D03	Melanoma in situ	M F	114 92	85 89	86 96	145 133	77 86	99 79	36 36	104 108	178 192

Table 6 Standardised registration ratios - *continued*

ICD (10th Revision) number	Site description		North East	North West	Yorkshire and the Humber	East Midlands	West Midlands	East of England	London	South East	South West
D04	Carcinoma in situ of skin	M	130	177	143	148	117	104	51	68	-
		F	156	184	159	124	125	101	36	63	-
D05	Carcinoma in situ of breast	M	569	131	176	268	-	-	-	70	-
		F	79	86	108	103	83	101	94	101	139
D06	Carcinoma in situ of cervix uteri	F	164	112	109	117	128	92	57	87	114
D07	Carcinoma in situ of other and unspecified genital organs	M	161	64	109	76	146	88	87	93	116
		F	100	140	93	115	105	78	59	80	146
D09	Carcinoma in situ of other and unspecified sites	M	272	149	191	27	29	65	109	90	46
		F	248	152	207	19	24	70	116	84	40
D33	Benign neoplasm of brain and other parts of central nervous system	M	148	56	85	108	63	103	58	140	170
		F	92	49	71	108	64	149	74	122	176
D35.2	Benign neoplasm of pituitary gland	M	76	105	138	160	115	84	105	112	-
		F	134	97	165	173	102	64	117	86	-
D35.3	Benign neoplasm of craniopharyngeal duct	M	-	-	-	-	-	-	-	-	-
		F	-	-	-	-	-	-	-	-	-
D35.4	Benign neoplasm of pineal gland	M	-	-	-	-	-	-	-	-	-
		F	-	-	-	-	-	-	-	-	-
D37	Neoplasm of uncertain or unknown behaviour of oral cavity and digestive organs	M	61	249	64	99	58	51	41	91	137
		F	107	178	59	126	57	47	43	123	139
D38	Neoplasm of uncertain or unknown behaviour of middle ear and respiratory and intrathoracic organs	M	-	167	56	16	39	25	-	168	306
		F	-	95	29	104	41	39	37	185	272
D39	Neoplasm of uncertain or unknown behaviour of female genital organs	F	57	132	36	121	75	120	48	91	215
D40	Neoplasm of uncertain or unknown behaviour of male genital organs	M	64	168	43	38	20	58	128	98	226
D41	Neoplasm of uncertain or unknown behaviour of urinary organs	M	-	11	51	176	222	130	3	94	198
		F	-	12	58	194	228	110	2	90	208
D42	Neoplasm of uncertain or unknown behaviour of meninges	M	105	121	-	126	463	-	45	33	51
		F	-	94	-	51	365	78	67	26	202
D43	Neoplasm of uncertain or unknown behaviour of brain and central nervous system	M	99	124	73	89	98	48	77	116	163
		F	46	122	79	76	147	69	68	103	153
D44	Neoplasm of uncertain or unknown behaviour of endocrine glands	M	43	106	88	64	82	39	26	121	298
		F	93	84	76	104	64	71	29	124	265
D45	Polycythaemia vera	M	29	59	80	160	125	66	83	191	49
		F	134	78	88	113	90	74	149	145	28
D46	Myelodysplastic syndromes	M	81	72	116	115	69	86	87	101	166
		F	67	83	108	140	58	76	72	96	192
D47	Other neoplasms of uncertain or unknown behaviour of lymphoid, haematopoietic and related tissue	M	69	43	193	64	43	82	104	147	126
		F	59	39	202	63	60	77	116	139	116
D48	Neoplasm of uncertain or unknown behaviour of other and unspecified sites	M	24	55	49	172	35	22	43	156	313
		F	26	107	24	103	46	44	60	143	292
O01	Hydatidiform mole	F	126	99	114	97	-	4	131	82	270

Table 9 Cancer mortality to incidence ratios: sex and government office for the region of residence, 2001

England, government offices for the regions Registered by May 2004

ICD (10th Revision) number	Site description	Sex	England	North East	North West	Yorkshire and the Humber	East Midlands	West Midlands	East of England	London	South East	South West
C00-C97	All cancers	M	0.47	0.49	0.48	0.46	0.46	0.46	0.50	0.58	0.48	0.39
		F	0.45	0.45	0.45	0.44	0.44	0.44	0.48	0.54	0.46	0.37
C00-C97 xC44	All cancers excluding nmsc	M	0.58	0.61	0.61	0.58	0.59	0.59	0.60	0.60	0.57	0.53
		F	0.54	0.57	0.57	0.54	0.54	0.55	0.56	0.55	0.54	0.48
C00-C14	Malignant neoplasm of lip, mouth and pharynx	M	0.39	0.40	0.41	0.44	0.33	0.38	0.36	0.42	0.35	0.42
		F	0.38	0.56	0.41	0.35	0.33	0.37	0.53	0.33	0.32	0.33
C00	Malignant neoplasm of lip	M	0.04	0.00	0.14	0.00	0.00	0.00	0.05	0.20	0.07	0.00
		F	0.06	0.00	0.13	0.00	0.00	0.00	0.10	0.00	0.13	0.25
C01	Malignant neoplasm of base of tongue	M	0.10	0.15	0.07	0.19	0.05	0.11	0.05	0.04	0.25	0.06
		F	0.11	0.33	0.17	0.14	0.00	0.11	0.00	0.11	0.13	0.00
C02	Malignant neoplasm of other and unspecified parts of tongue	M	0.49	0.38	0.53	0.52	0.29	0.41	0.53	0.58	0.55	0.43
		F	0.47	1.60	0.45	0.54	0.38	0.23	0.74	0.43	0.43	0.47
C03	Malignant neoplasm of gum	M	0.35	3.00	0.45	1.20	0.25	0.44	0.23	0.21	0.16	0.50
		F	0.36	1.50	0.50	0.14	0.08	0.50	0.67	0.09	0.38	0.33
C04	Malignant neoplasm of floor of mouth	M	0.19	0.14	0.20	0.28	0.19	0.19	0.31	0.12	0.14	0.13
		F	0.18	0.00	0.19	0.11	0.08	0.18	0.44	0.15	0.21	0.17
C05	Malignant neoplasm of palate	M	0.30	0.38	0.27	0.50	0.27	0.50	0.14	0.54	0.29	0.00
		F	0.24	0.18	0.36	0.21	0.40	0.83	0.13	0.22	0.06	0.13
C06	Malignant neoplasm of other and unspecified parts of mouth	M	0.50	1.00	0.52	0.35	0.79	0.83	0.47	0.55	0.21	0.45
		F	0.56	1.33	0.46	0.67	0.38	0.69	0.78	0.55	0.41	0.54
C07	Malignant neoplasm of parotid gland	M	0.39	1.00	0.26	0.48	0.33	0.35	0.47	0.35	0.23	0.52
		F	0.39	0.40	0.29	0.22	0.23	0.65	1.08	0.19	0.50	0.22
C08	Malignant neoplasm of other and unspecified major salivary glands	M	0.33	0.50	0.57	0.00	0.29	0.00	0.00	0.43	0.36	0.57
		F	0.22	0.00	0.57	0.00	0.00	0.00	0.25	0.33	0.00	0.57
C09	Malignant neoplasm of tonsil	M	0.37	0.43	0.38	0.30	0.40	0.49	0.23	0.38	0.35	0.43
		F	0.34	1.00	0.47	0.17	0.60	0.25	0.25	0.25	0.06	0.50
C10	Malignant neoplasm of oropharynx	M	0.74	0.13	1.10	1.90	0.50	0.18	0.67	0.60	0.46	1.50
		F	1.03	1.00	1.00	1.67	2.00	0.50	0.75	0.75	1.25	0.33
C11	Malignant neoplasm of nasopharynx	M	0.52	0.50	0.70	0.83	0.25	0.58	0.29	0.75	0.83	0.29
		F	0.28	-	0.27	0.80	0.00	0.33	0.00	0.27	0.29	0.09
C12	Malignant neoplasm of piriform sinus	M	0.31	0.14	0.17	0.26	0.10	0.25	0.44	0.53	0.41	0.71
		F	0.25	0.67	0.29	0.00	0.00	0.40	0.00	0.40	0.00	0.33
C13	Malignant neoplasm of hypopharynx	M	0.55	0.29	0.35	0.09	2.25	0.64	1.00	0.33	0.42	1.75
		F	0.43	0.40	0.79	0.22	0.57	0.50	0.50	0.29	0.13	0.29
C14	Malignant neoplasm of other and ill-defined sites in the lip, oral cavity and pharynx	M	1.00	2.25	0.93	2.00	0.54	1.25	2.00	0.52	0.88	0.92
		F	0.72	-	0.50	0.50	1.33	2.00	1.00	0.58	0.71	0.50
C15	Malignant neoplasm of oesophagus	M	0.95	1.12	0.98	0.95	0.88	0.94	1.10	1.01	0.92	0.84
		F	0.90	0.85	0.95	1.01	0.90	0.89	0.93	0.86	0.80	0.89
C16	Malignant neoplasm of stomach	M	0.68	0.65	0.66	0.73	0.68	0.65	0.70	0.67	0.71	0.65
		F	0.75	0.75	0.74	0.70	0.75	0.88	0.65	0.79	0.78	0.73
C17	Malignant neoplasm of small intestine	M	0.41	0.28	0.43	0.39	0.53	0.33	0.43	0.50	0.45	0.32
		F	0.44	0.18	0.56	0.63	0.35	0.35	0.55	0.48	0.39	0.34
C18-C20	Malignant neoplasm of colon and rectum	M	0.46	0.47	0.47	0.44	0.45	0.45	0.46	0.48	0.51	0.45
		F	0.48	0.47	0.48	0.46	0.47	0.51	0.48	0.49	0.51	0.44
C18	Malignant neoplasm of colon	M	0.50	0.51	0.51	0.51	0.47	0.49	0.50	0.54	0.56	0.45
		F	0.50	0.48	0.48	0.51	0.49	0.51	0.52	0.53	0.53	0.44
C19	Malignant neoplasm of rectosigmoid junction	M	0.35	0.39	0.30	0.24	0.30	0.48	0.42	0.41	0.32	0.45
		F	0.36	0.42	0.37	0.30	0.48	0.45	0.28	0.34	0.47	0.18

Table 9 Cancer mortality to incidence ratios - *continued*

ICD (10th Revision) number	Site description		England	North East	North West	Yorkshire and the Humber	East Midlands	West Midlands	East of England	London	South East	South West
C20	Malignant neoplasm of rectum	M	**0.42**	0.43	0.44	0.39	0.44	0.37	0.39	0.38	0.47	0.47
		F	**0.46**	0.48	0.53	0.40	0.41	0.50	0.43	0.46	0.46	0.49
C21	Malignant neoplasm of anus and anal canal	M	**0.28**	0.33	0.32	0.22	0.24	0.58	0.21	0.19	0.26	0.35
		F	**0.30**	0.24	0.31	0.50	0.48	0.30	0.42	0.22	0.25	0.26
C22	Malignant neoplasm of liver and intrahepatic bile ducts	M	**0.89**	0.82	0.77	0.93	1.00	0.85	1.12	0.87	0.88	0.91
		F	**0.92**	0.97	0.60	1.01	0.94	0.98	1.27	1.00	1.22	0.89
C23	Malignant neoplasm of gallbladder	M	**0.69**	0.71	1.25	0.88	0.50	0.57	0.69	0.25	0.63	1.11
		F	**0.77**	0.77	0.67	0.72	0.90	0.74	0.85	0.71	0.77	0.97
C24	Malignant neoplasm of other and unspecified parts of biliary tract	M	**0.28**	0.47	0.39	0.29	0.27	0.22	0.24	0.28	0.26	0.23
		F	**0.28**	0.29	0.54	0.42	0.41	0.60	0.42	0.14	0.08	0.10
C25	Malignant neoplasm of pancreas	M	**0.97**	0.86	1.08	0.91	0.84	0.94	1.15	0.95	0.95	0.96
		F	**0.99**	0.92	1.06	0.90	0.99	1.06	0.93	0.97	1.04	0.99
C26	Malignant neoplasm of other and ill-defined digestive organs	M	**4.11**	22.33	4.32	7.00	3.70	10.00	10.27	2.92	2.24	2.00
		F	**2.95**	26.00	3.51	6.36	4.10	8.40	3.69	2.02	1.60	1.78
C30	Malignant neoplasm of nasal cavity and middle ear	M	**0.12**	0.00	0.00	0.25	0.40	0.17	0.06	0.33	0.09	0.00
		F	**0.14**	0.00	0.07	0.29	0.33	0.00	0.00	0.50	0.13	0.15
C31	Malignant neoplasm of accessory sinuses	M	**0.59**	0.75	0.64	0.30	1.00	0.38	0.63	0.50	0.75	0.50
		F	**0.83**	1.50	0.58	-	1.00	0.67	0.25	0.89	1.00	1.29
C32	Malignant neoplasm of larynx	M	**0.39**	0.42	0.43	0.37	0.33	0.45	0.36	0.39	0.36	0.32
		F	**0.41**	0.54	0.38	0.21	0.31	0.71	0.56	0.26	0.56	0.35
C33-C34	Malignant neoplasm of trachea, bronchus and lung	M	**0.89**	0.90	0.90	0.91	0.87	0.92	0.87	0.89	0.88	0.84
		F	**0.87**	0.88	0.88	0.87	0.85	0.89	0.90	0.85	0.88	0.85
C33	Malignant neoplasm of trachea	M	**0.47**	1.00	0.50	0.50	0.25	0.25	0.50	1.00	0.43	1.00
		F	**0.57**	2.00	0.44	0.50	0.00	1.00	0.00	0.50	1.50	0.50
C34	Malignant neoplasm of bronchus and lung	M	**0.89**	0.90	0.90	0.91	0.87	0.92	0.87	0.89	0.88	0.84
		F	**0.87**	0.88	0.88	0.87	0.85	0.89	0.90	0.85	0.88	0.85
C37	Malignant neoplasm of thymus	M	**0.40**	0.50	1.00	0.14	1.00	0.33	0.00	0.00	0.00	0.80
			0.33	0.00	0.00	1.00	0.00	0.40	0.25	0.25	2.00	0.40
C38	Malignant neoplasm of heart, mediastinum and pleura	M	**0.41**	0.50	0.21	0.31	0.56	0.50	0.57	1.14	0.29	0.45
		F	**0.41**	3.00	0.22	0.27	1.00	0.50	0.50	0.50	0.67	0.11
C39	Malignant neoplasm of other and ill-defined sites in the respiratory system and intrathoracic organs	M	**4.25**	-	-	-	-	-	-	0.67	-	0.00
		F	**2.67**	-	4.00	-	-	0.00	0.00	-	-	-
C40	Malignant neoplasm of bone and articular cartilage of limbs	M	**0.21**	0.13	0.12	0.38	0.00	0.27	0.50	0.24	0.20	0.09
		F	**0.20**	0.33	0.25	0.20	0.25	0.15	0.33	0.23	0.14	0.13
C41	Malignant neoplasm of bone and articular cartilage of other and unspecified sites	M	**0.98**	2.00	0.35	1.29	0.88	2.00	0.73	1.36	1.40	0.76
		F	**0.84**	1.00	0.31	2.17	0.73	1.20	1.17	1.11	1.13	0.69
C43	Malignant melanoma of skin	M	**0.27**	0.30	0.29	0.24	0.31	0.26	0.31	0.37	0.26	0.21
		F	**0.19**	0.17	0.21	0.13	0.16	0.18	0.21	0.33	0.23	0.14
C44	Other malignant neoplasms of skin	M	**0.01**	0.01	0.01	0.01	0.00	0.01	0.01	0.05	0.01	0.01
		F	**0.01**	0.01	0.01	0.01	0.01	0.01	0.01	0.05	0.01	0.00
C45	Mesothelioma	M	**0.90**	1.06	0.82	0.84	0.91	0.68	0.89	1.04	0.93	0.90
		F	**0.71**	0.68	1.11	0.79	0.69	0.67	0.66	0.60	0.63	0.66
C46	Kaposi's sarcoma	M	**0.06**	0.00	0.00	0.00	0.00	0.00	0.00	0.09	0.13	0.00
		F	**0.06**	-	0.00	-	-	-	0.00	0.07	-	-
C47	Malignant neoplasm of peripheral nerves and autonomic nervous system	M	**0.33**	0.50	0.50	0.25	0.17	0.17	0.33	0.67	0.25	0.43
		F	**0.33**	0.00	0.40	0.50	0.60	0.17	0.67	1.00	0.00	0.17
C48	Malignant neoplasm of retroperitoneum and peritoneum	M	**0.47**	0.00	0.41	0.75	0.29	0.27	0.67	1.10	0.45	0.17
		F	**0.52**	0.35	0.61	0.80	0.25	0.63	0.50	0.48	0.55	0.68

Table 9 Cancer mortality to incidence ratios - *continued*

ICD (10th Revision) number	Site description		England	North East	North West	Yorkshire and the Humber	East Midlands	West Midlands	East of England	London	South East	South West
C49	Malignant neoplasm of other connective and soft tissue	M F	**0.49** **0.54**	0.58 0.63	0.24 0.61	0.50 0.54	0.27 0.52	0.70 0.45	0.57 0.55	1.03 0.79	0.60 0.59	0.34 0.35
C50	Malignant neoplasm of breast	M F	**0.32** **0.32**	0.13 0.32	0.34 0.32	0.57 0.31	2.50 0.34	0.29 0.30	0.17 0.33	0.30 0.33	0.22 0.31	0.21 0.29
C51	Malignant neoplasm of vulva	F	**0.38**	0.28	0.38	0.36	0.34	0.40	0.46	0.59	0.45	0.20
C52	Malignant neoplasm of vagina	F	**0.39**	0.29	0.37	0.36	0.40	0.41	0.45	0.55	0.49	0.22
C53	Malignant neoplasm of cervix uteri	F	**0.39**	0.43	0.40	0.36	0.35	0.36	0.40	0.46	0.43	0.35
C54	Malignant neoplasm of corpus uteri	F	**0.18**	0.17	0.20	0.17	0.14	0.20	0.16	0.19	0.21	0.18
C55	Malignant neoplasm of uterus, part unspecified	F	**1.59**	1.15	1.10	1.16	1.29	1.65	2.42	2.04	1.66	2.84
C56-C57	Malignant neoplasm of ovary and other unspecified female genital organs	F	**0.68**	0.60	0.68	0.63	0.63	0.67	0.74	0.67	0.72	0.67
C56	Malignant neoplasm of ovary	F	**0.67**	0.60	0.67	0.63	0.62	0.66	0.74	0.67	0.72	0.67
C57	Malignant neoplasm of other and unspecified female genital organs	F	**0.68**	0.60	0.68	0.63	0.63	0.67	0.75	0.68	0.71	0.66
C58	Malignant neoplasm of placenta	F	**0.33**	-	1.00	-	-	0.00	0.00	1.00	0.00	-
C60	Malignant neoplasm of penis	M	**0.26**	0.14	0.31	0.15	0.28	0.32	0.20	0.35	0.30	0.25
C61	Malignant neoplasm of prostate	M	**0.32**	0.28	0.33	0.30	0.35	0.32	0.33	0.32	0.32	0.31
C62	Malignant neoplasm of testis	M	**0.03**	0.00	0.05	0.02	0.06	0.03	0.04	0.02	0.03	0.04
C63	Malignant neoplasm of other and unspecified male genital organs	M	**0.17**	0.67	0.11	0.00	0.25	0.10	0.00	0.20	0.33	0.20
C64	Malignant neoplasm of kidney, except renal pelvis	M F	**0.56** **0.59**	0.60 0.59	0.63 0.64	0.56 0.47	0.46 0.68	0.63 0.57	0.62 0.58	0.56 0.56	0.51 0.67	0.50 0.51
C65	Malignant neoplasm of renal pelvis	M F	**0.05** **0.07**	0.04 0.00	0.04 0.06	0.11 0.04	0.00 0.09	0.06 0.00	0.06 0.09	0.00 0.33	0.09 0.06	0.00 0.17
C66	Malignant neoplasm of ureter	M F	**0.30** **0.30**	0.19 0.00	0.20 0.29	0.36 0.21	0.23 0.17	0.16 0.50	0.67 0.40	0.38 0.20	0.38 1.00	0.22 0.33
C67	Malignant neoplasm of bladder	M F	**0.44** **0.55**	0.45 0.52	0.34 0.52	0.45 0.50	0.42 0.46	0.50 0.64	0.50 0.62	0.49 0.56	0.48 0.62	0.38 0.53
C68	Malignant neoplasm of other and unspecified urinery organs	M F	**0.67** **0.39**	1.00 0.00	0.28 0.00	0.33 1.00	0.70 0.25	1.17 0.33	1.11 0.20	0.63 1.00	1.00 0.17	0.50 1.00
C69	Malignant neoplasm of eye and adnexa	M F	**0.16** **0.21**	0.50 0.00	0.10 0.38	0.10 0.43	0.19 0.08	0.26 0.38	0.42 0.36	0.18 0.18	0.11 0.18	0.05 0.10
C70	Malignant neoplasm of meninges	M F	**0.60** **0.16**	0.00 -	0.60 0.09	3.00 0.60	0.33 0.00	0.50 2.00	0.50 0.00	0.33 0.00	1.00 0.14	0.50 0.33
C71	Malignant neoplasm of brain	M F	**0.80** **0.77**	0.74 0.79	0.76 0.64	0.72 0.78	0.84 0.79	0.77 1.02	0.88 0.85	0.85 0.63	0.77 0.81	0.85 0.74
C72	Malignant neoplasm of spinal cord, cranial nerves and other parts of central nervous system	M F	**0.16** **0.17**	0.00 0.50	0.50 0.25	0.00 0.25	0.75 0.20	0.20 0.14	0.11 0.14	0.25 0.00	0.00 0.25	0.13 0.00
C73	Malignant neoplasm of thyroid gland	M F	**0.24** **0.19**	0.38 0.14	0.22 0.28	0.21 0.17	0.33 0.17	0.21 0.15	0.29 0.21	0.24 0.14	0.23 0.20	0.16 0.23
C74	Malignant neoplasm of adrenal gland	M F	**0.67** **0.49**	0.14 0.71	0.63 0.40	0.60 0.83	0.33 0.30	1.40 0.38	0.78 0.89	1.00 0.67	0.71 0.28	0.60 0.38
C75	Malignant neoplasm of other endocrine glands and related structures	M F	**0.49** **0.44**	0.00 0.00	0.33 1.50	0.43 0.40	1.00 2.00	1.50 0.75	0.33 1.33	1.00 0.00	0.83 0.00	0.11 0.14

Table 9 Cancer mortality to incidence ratios - *continued*

ICD (10th Revision) number	Site description		England	North East	North West	Yorkshire and the Humber	East Midlands	West Midlands	East of England	London	South East	South West
C76	Malignant neoplasm of other and ill-defined sites	M F	**0.86** **0.81**	3.00 2.17	1.21 1.20	2.83 2.46	1.69 1.60	3.40 1.44	0.96 0.72	0.32 0.28	0.50 0.69	0.69 0.74
C77	Secondary and unspecified malignant neoplasm of lymph nodes	M F	**0.01** **0.02**	0.00 0.12	0.03 0.02	0.00 0.00	0.00 0.00	0.00 0.00	0.00 0.03	0.00 0.00	0.00 0.05	0.00 0.00
C78	Secondary malignant neoplasm of respiratory and digestive organs	M F	**0.24** **0.22**	0.22 0.15	0.34 0.45	0.15 0.23	0.17 0.15	0.36 0.28	0.23 0.26	0.17 0.23	0.24 0.17	0.29 0.12
C79	Secondary malignant neoplasm of other sites	M F	**0.26** **0.30**	0.32 0.30	0.63 0.67	0.23 0.23	0.20 0.28	0.24 0.37	0.25 0.33	0.26 0.15	0.26 0.20	0.14 0.35
C80	Malignant neoplasm without specification of site	M F	**2.11** **1.91**	3.03 2.26	1.55 1.53	2.37 2.10	3.57 2.68	1.77 1.59	2.39 1.93	2.25 1.94	2.32 2.13	1.70 1.79
C81	Hodgkin's disease	M F	**0.18** **0.18**	0.22 0.16	0.16 0.19	0.13 0.27	0.18 0.26	0.25 0.16	0.27 0.13	0.16 0.17	0.15 0.17	0.14 0.15
C82-C85	Non-Hodgkin's lymphoma	M F	**0.49** **0.50**	0.50 0.47	0.55 0.57	0.41 0.46	0.42 0.49	0.52 0.54	0.53 0.54	0.55 0.51	0.49 0.52	0.41 0.39
C82	Follicular (nodular) non-Hodgkin's lymphoma	M F	**0.04** **0.04**	0.00 0.00	0.01 0.04	0.10 0.13	0.04 0.04	0.00 0.02	0.02 0.02	0.06 0.04	0.02 0.06	0.06 0.03
C83	Diffuse non-Hodgkin's lymphoma lymphoma	M F	**0.07** **0.06**	0.02 0.08	0.04 0.10	0.08 0.06	0.08 0.05	0.05 0.04	0.12 0.04	0.11 0.05	0.09 0.05	0.07 0.06
C84	Peripheral and cutaneous T-cell lymphomas	M F	**0.40** **0.40**	0.43 0.25	0.68 0.47	0.21 0.24	0.41 0.43	0.15 0.22	0.22 0.67	0.74 0.71	0.60 0.45	0.41 0.42
C85	Other and unspecified types on non-Hodgkin's lymphoma	M F	**0.95** **0.96**	1.29 1.15	1.00 0.99	0.97 1.15	1.00 1.10	1.43 1.45	0.88 0.81	0.79 0.75	1.01 1.08	0.76 0.71
C88	Malignant immunoproliferative diseases	M F	**0.44** **0.65**	0.75 1.00	0.67 1.00	0.67 0.63	0.63 0.38	0.78 1.40	1.25 0.80	0.25 1.13	0.35 0.44	0.14 0.50
C90	Multiple myeloma and malignant plasma cell neoplasms	M F	**0.69** **0.77**	0.64 0.98	0.85 0.88	0.59 0.68	0.73 0.91	0.80 0.86	0.78 0.86	0.72 0.64	0.57 0.66	0.63 0.74
C91-C95	All leukaemias	M F	**0.62** **0.64**	0.74 0.63	0.80 0.75	0.49 0.55	0.60 0.77	0.65 0.63	0.69 0.74	0.59 0.69	0.57 0.60	0.60 0.55
C91	Lymphoid leukaemia	M F	**0.43** **0.41**	0.63 0.43	0.67 0.61	0.32 0.29	0.42 0.51	0.45 0.45	0.52 0.58	0.41 0.44	0.35 0.35	0.38 0.31
C92	Myeloid leukaemia	M F	**0.82** **0.87**	0.80 0.82	0.91 0.84	0.71 0.86	0.78 0.91	0.91 0.86	0.79 0.84	0.76 0.89	0.81 0.89	0.92 0.86
C93	Monocytic leukaemia	M F	**0.29** **0.23**	- 1.00	- -	0.00 0.40	0.50 0.00	0.43 0.14	0.33 0.00	0.08 0.25	0.23 0.11	0.33 0.40
C94	Other leukaemias of specified cell type	M F	**0.33** **0.91**	1.00 0.50	0.50 0.00	1.00 -	0.00 -	0.25 0.33	0.00 -	0.20 3.00	0.00 0.50	1.00 -
C95	Leukaemia of unspecified cell type	M F	**1.19** **0.98**	1.50 0.63	0.88 0.88	1.67 1.25	2.00 1.33	0.75 0.80	1.64 1.38	2.00 1.22	1.27 1.06	0.71 0.67
C96	Other and unspecified malignant neoplasms of lymphoid, haematopoietic and related tissue	M F	**0.26** **0.27**	- -	- -	0.00 -	1.00 0.50	0.50 0.50	0.33 0.50	0.00 0.00	0.00 0.00	0.50 0.00
C97	Malignant neoplasms of independent(primary) multiple sites	M F	- -	- -	- -	- -	- -	- -	- -	- -	- -	- -

Table 10 Directly age standardised* registration rates per 100,000 population: site and sex, 1992 to 2001 — **England**

ICD (10th Revision) number	Site description		1992	1993	1994	1995	1996	1997	1998	1999	2000	2001
	All registrations	M	480.9	477.3	487.8	499.0	494.5	508.6	517.9	519.8	536.3	535.8
		F	475.7	462.0	473.1	487.5	491.9	510.4	524.5	531.0	529.1	526.0
C00-C97	All cancers	M	463.1	457.7	466.8	473.5	467.0	478.3	487.2	485.5	495.3	494.3
		F	375.1	363.1	368.8	376.4	375.8	392.7	398.0	403.1	401.8	401.3
C00-C97 xC44	All cancers excluding nmsc	M	394.3	391.5	398.0	401.3	395.1	397.6	395.6	395.8	401.4	399.5
		F	328.5	320.5	323.8	328.7	327.5	339.1	337.8	342.8	338.4	336.9
C00-C14	Malignant neoplasm of lip, mouth and pharynx	M	8.7	8.4	8.9	8.6	8.8	9.1	9.2	10.0	10.1	10.0
		F	3.9	3.7	3.8	3.9	4.0	4.5	4.3	4.5	4.7	4.6
C00	Malignant neoplasm of lip	M	0.7	0.6	0.7	0.6	0.7	0.6	0.5	0.6	0.6	0.6
		F	0.2	0.1	0.2	0.1	0.2	0.2	0.2	0.2	0.3	0.2
C01	Malignant neoplasm of base of tongue	M	0.4	0.3	0.5	0.4	0.4	0.4	0.5	0.6	0.6	0.7
		F	0.1	0.2	0.1	0.1	0.1	0.1	0.2	0.2	0.2	0.2
C02	Malignant neoplasm of other and unspecified parts of tongue	M	1.4	1.5	1.5	1.4	1.5	1.6	1.6	1.7	1.7	1.7
		F	0.8	0.8	0.7	0.7	0.8	1.0	0.9	1.0	0.9	1.0
C03	Malignant neoplasm of gum	M	0.3	0.2	0.3	0.2	0.3	0.3	0.2	0.3	0.4	0.4
		F	0.2	0.2	0.2	0.2	0.2	0.2	0.2	0.2	0.3	0.3
C04	Malignant neoplasm of floor of mouth	M	0.9	0.9	0.9	0.9	0.9	0.8	0.9	0.9	0.9	1.0
		F	0.3	0.3	0.3	0.3	0.3	0.3	0.3	0.3	0.3	0.3
C05	Malignant neoplasm of palate	M	0.5	0.4	0.4	0.4	0.4	0.5	0.5	0.5	0.5	0.5
		F	0.2	0.3	0.3	0.2	0.2	0.3	0.3	0.2	0.3	0.3
C06	Malignant neoplasm of other and unspecified parts of mouth	M	0.7	0.6	0.7	0.6	0.7	0.7	0.7	0.7	0.7	0.8
		F	0.4	0.3	0.4	0.5	0.4	0.5	0.5	0.5	0.5	0.4
C07	Malignant neoplasm of parotid gland	M	0.6	0.6	0.7	0.7	0.6	0.6	0.7	0.6	0.6	0.7
		F	0.5	0.3	0.4	0.5	0.4	0.5	0.4	0.4	0.4	0.5
C08	Malignant neoplasm of other and unspecified major salivary glands	M	0.2	0.2	0.2	0.2	0.2	0.2	0.3	0.2	0.2	0.2
		F	0.1	0.1	0.2	0.1	0.2	0.2	0.2	0.2	0.2	0.2
C09	Malignant neoplasm of tonsil	M	0.9	0.8	0.8	0.9	1.0	1.1	1.2	1.3	1.4	1.3
		F	0.3	0.3	0.3	0.3	0.3	0.4	0.4	0.4	0.5	0.4
C10	Malignant neoplasm of oropharynx	M	0.3	0.4	0.4	0.4	0.4	0.3	0.3	0.4	0.4	0.4
		F	0.1	0.1	0.1	0.1	0.1	0.1	0.1	0.1	0.1	0.1
C11	Malignant neoplasm of nasopharynx	M	0.5	0.5	0.5	0.5	0.6	0.5	0.5	0.6	0.5	0.4
		F	0.2	0.2	0.2	0.2	0.3	0.2	0.2	0.2	0.3	0.2
C12	Malignant neoplasm of pyriform sinus	M	0.7	0.7	0.6	0.7	0.6	0.6	0.7	0.8	0.8	0.6
		F	0.2	0.1	0.1	0.1	0.1	0.2	0.1	0.1	0.1	0.1
C13	Malignant neoplasm of hypopharynx	M	0.3	0.3	0.3	0.3	0.2	0.3	0.3	0.3	0.3	0.3
		F	0.2	0.2	0.2	0.2	0.2	0.2	0.2	0.2	0.1	0.2
C14	Malignant neoplasm of other and ill-defined sites in the lip, oral cavity and pharynx	M	0.4	0.4	0.5	0.5	0.5	0.4	0.5	0.5	0.5	0.4
		F	0.2	0.2	0.2	0.2	0.2	0.2	0.2	0.2	0.2	0.2
C15	Malignant neoplasm of oesophagus	M	12.4	12.5	12.9	12.6	12.7	13.0	12.8	13.0	13.4	13.6
		F	5.7	5.5	5.8	5.7	5.4	5.6	5.6	5.9	5.7	5.6
C16	Malignant neoplasm of stomach	M	22.4	21.1	21.0	20.3	19.6	19.7	18.9	18.4	17.6	16.4
		F	8.8	8.3	8.2	8.0	7.5	7.8	7.3	6.7	6.9	6.5
C17	Malignant neoplasm of small intestine	M	0.9	0.8	0.9	0.9	1.0	1.0	1.2	1.2	1.2	1.2
		F	0.6	0.5	0.6	0.6	0.7	0.7	0.7	0.8	0.8	0.8
C18-C21	Malignant neoplasm of colon, rectum and anus	M	53.8	53.5	52.6	53.4	55.0	55.6	56.0	55.6	55.5	53.1
		F	37.1	35.4	35.5	35.1	36.3	35.8	37.1	36.7	35.4	34.5
C18-C20	Malignant neoplasm of colon and rectum	M	52.9	52.6	51.8	52.5	54.1	54.6	55.0	54.6	54.6	52.2
		F	36.1	34.5	34.6	34.1	35.3	34.6	36.0	35.5	34.2	33.4

* Using the European standard population

Table 10 Directly age standardised* rates - *continued*   **England**

ICD (10th Revision) number	Site description		1992	1993	1994	1995	1996	1997	1998	1999	2000	2001
C18	Malignant neoplasm of colon	M	30.8	31.2	30.7	31.8	32.0	32.4	31.7	31.7	31.8	30.8
		F	24.8	23.4	23.7	23.5	24.1	23.4	24.0	23.5	23.2	22.5
C19	Malignant neoplasm of rectosigmoid junction	M	3.9	3.7	4.0	3.8	4.2	4.3	4.6	4.7	4.4	4.3
		F	2.1	2.1	2.2	2.2	2.4	2.5	2.5	2.7	2.5	2.3
C20	Malignant neoplasm of rectum	M	18.1	17.6	17.0	16.9	17.9	17.9	18.8	18.3	18.4	17.1
		F	9.2	9.0	8.6	8.4	8.9	8.8	9.4	9.3	8.5	8.5
C21	Malignant neoplasm of anus and anal canal	M	0.9	0.9	0.8	0.9	0.9	1.0	0.9	1.0	1.0	0.9
		F	1.0	1.0	0.9	1.0	1.0	1.2	1.2	1.2	1.2	1.2
C22	Malignant neoplasm of liver and intrahepatic bile ducts	M	3.2	3.2	3.4	3.6	4.0	4.1	4.3	4.2	4.8	4.5
		F	1.4	1.4	1.6	1.7	2.0	2.1	2.1	2.0	2.2	2.3
C23	Malignant neoplasm of gallbladder	M	0.6	0.4	0.4	0.5	0.4	0.4	0.4	0.5	0.4	0.4
		F	0.9	0.9	0.9	0.7	0.8	0.8	0.8	0.8	0.8	0.8
C24	Malignant neoplasm of other and unspecified parts of biliary tract	M	1.6	1.4	1.2	1.2	1.3	1.1	1.1	1.1	1.1	1.0
		F	1.0	1.0	0.9	0.9	0.9	0.7	0.9	0.9	0.9	0.8
C25	Malignant neoplasm of pancreas	M	11.0	10.6	10.2	10.4	10.3	10.2	10.2	10.2	10.4	10.0
		F	7.8	7.8	7.8	7.7	7.6	7.4	7.2	7.9	7.8	7.4
C26	Malignant neoplasm of other and ill-defined digestive organs	M	1.0	0.8	0.9	0.9	1.0	1.1	1.0	1.0	0.9	0.8
		F	0.7	0.6	0.6	0.6	0.6	0.8	0.6	0.8	0.6	0.7
C30	Malignant neoplasm of nasal cavity and middle ear	M	0.4	0.4	0.4	0.3	0.4	0.4	0.4	0.3	0.5	0.4
		F	0.3	0.3	0.2	0.2	0.2	0.2	0.2	0.3	0.3	0.3
C31	Malignant neoplasm of accessory sinuses	M	0.5	0.4	0.3	0.4	0.4	0.3	0.4	0.3	0.3	0.3
		F	0.2	0.2	0.2	0.2	0.2	0.2	0.2	0.2	0.2	0.2
C32	Malignant neoplasm of larynx	M	6.2	6.0	6.4	5.8	5.8	5.9	5.6	5.5	6.0	5.5
		F	1.1	1.2	1.1	1.1	1.0	1.1	1.0	1.0	1.0	1.0
C33-C34	Malignant neoplasm of trachea, bronchus and lung	M	89.1	83.3	82.2	79.2	74.9	73.8	71.0	68.9	67.4	64.8
		F	33.9	33.2	33.6	33.8	33.1	33.2	33.7	33.6	34.0	33.3
C33	Malignant neoplasm of trachea	M	0.2	0.2	0.2	0.2	0.1	0.2	0.1	0.1	0.1	0.1
		F	0.1	0.2	0.1	0.1	0.1	0.1	0.1	0.1	0.1	0.1
C34	Malignant neoplasm of bronchus and lung	M	89.0	83.1	82.0	79.1	74.8	73.6	70.9	68.8	67.3	64.7
		F	33.8	33.1	33.5	33.7	33.0	33.2	33.7	33.5	33.9	33.2
C37	Malignant neoplasm of thymus	M	0.1	0.1	0.1	0.1	0.1	0.1	0.1	0.1	0.1	0.1
		F	0.1	0.1	0.1	0.1	0.1	0.1	0.1	0.1	0.1	0.1
C38	Malignant neoplasm of heart, mediastinum and pleura	M	0.9	0.8	0.6	0.8	0.6	0.7	0.6	0.7	0.7	0.5
		F	0.3	0.4	0.3	0.4	0.3	0.4	0.3	0.3	0.3	0.3
C39	Malignant neoplasm of other and ill-defined sites in the respiratory system and intrathoracic organs	M	0.0	0.0	0.0	0.0	0.0	0.0	0.0	0.0	0.0	0.0
		F	0.0	0.0	0.0	0.0	0.0	0.0	0.0	0.0	0.0	0.0
C40	Malignant neoplasm of bone and articular cartilage of limbs	M	0.4	0.4	0.4	0.5	0.4	0.5	0.5	0.4	0.5	0.5
		F	0.2	0.3	0.3	0.3	0.4	0.3	0.4	0.4	0.3	0.3
C41	Malignant neoplasm of bone and articular cartilage of other and unspecified sites	M	0.5	0.3	0.4	0.5	0.4	0.4	0.4	0.5	0.5	0.4
		F	0.3	0.3	0.3	0.3	0.4	0.3	0.3	0.3	0.3	0.4
C43	Malignant melanoma of skin	M	6.4	7.3	7.3	7.6	7.5	8.3	8.6	8.4	9.7	10.0
		F	8.4	9.6	9.4	9.9	9.5	9.8	9.9	9.9	11.2	11.7
C44	Other malignant neoplasms of skin	M	68.8	66.2	68.8	72.2	72.0	80.7	91.6	89.8	93.9	94.8
		F	46.6	42.6	45.0	47.7	48.3	53.6	60.2	60.7	63.3	64.4
C45	Mesothelioma	M	3.3	3.6	3.6	3.9	3.8	4.1	4.7	4.7	5.0	5.1
		F	0.5	0.5	0.5	0.5	0.5	0.6	0.6	0.7	0.7	0.9
C46	Kaposi's sarcoma	M	0.6	0.7	0.6	0.6	0.4	0.3	0.3	0.2	0.2	0.2
		F	0.1	0.0	0.1	0.1	0.0	0.0	0.0	0.0	0.0	0.1

* Using the European standard population

Table 10 Directly age standardised* rates - continued

England

ICD (10th Revision) number	Site description		1992	1993	1994	1995	1996	1997	1998	1999	2000	2001
C47	Malignant neoplasm of peripheral nerves and autonomic nervous system	M F	0.2 0.1	0.1 0.2	0.1 0.2	0.2 0.2	0.2 0.2	0.2 0.2	0.2 0.2	0.2 0.2	0.2 0.2	0.2 0.2
C48	Malignant neoplasm of retroperitoneum and peritoneum	M F	0.4 0.4	0.5 0.4	0.6 0.4	0.4 0.5	0.4 0.5	0.4 0.5	0.3 0.6	0.3 0.6	0.5 0.6	0.4 0.6
C49	Malignant neoplasm of other connective and soft tissue	M F	2.6 2.0	2.2 1.6	2.2 1.5	1.8 1.4	2.1 1.5	2.0 1.5	2.3 1.4	2.1 1.6	2.2 1.5	2.0 1.5
C50	Malignant neoplasm of breast	M F	0.7 106.4	0.9 101.4	0.7 103.5	0.8 105.7	0.7 106.4	0.9 113.2	1.0 113.4	1.0 116.7	0.7 114.0	0.9 114.6
C51	Malignant neoplasm of vulva	F	2.3	2.1	2.2	2.1	2.1	2.1	2.2	2.3	2.2	2.3
C52	Malignant neoplasm of vagina	F	0.5	0.6	0.5	0.5	0.5	0.5	0.5	0.6	0.5	0.5
C53	Malignant neoplasm of cervix uteri	F	11.8	11.5	11.0	10.4	10.0	9.7	9.2	9.4	8.6	8.6
C54	Malignant neoplasm of corpus uteri	F	12.4	12.7	12.8	13.0	13.0	13.8	13.5	14.1	15.4	15.1
C55	Malignant neoplasm of uterus, part unspecified	F	1.2	0.8	0.8	0.9	0.8	0.9	1.0	0.9	0.8	0.8
C56-C57	Malignant neoplasm of ovary and other and unspecified female genital organs	F	17.4	16.9	16.9	18.6	18.4	19.3	19.1	18.3	17.9	18.4
C56	Malignant neoplasm of ovary	F	17.0	16.7	16.7	18.2	18.1	18.8	18.7	17.9	17.5	18.1
C57	Malignant neoplasm of other and unspecified female genital organs	F	0.4	0.2	0.2	0.4	0.4	0.5	0.4	0.4	0.4	0.3
C58	Malignant neoplasm of placenta	F	0.0	0.0	0.0	0.0	0.0	0.0	0.0	0.0	0.0	0.0
C60	Malignant neoplasm of penis	M	1.1	1.2	1.2	1.2	1.2	1.2	1.2	1.1	1.4	1.2
C61	Malignant neoplasm of prostate	M	54.4	58.5	66.1	68.8	68.7	67.3	68.8	72.9	80.4	89.8
C62	Malignant neoplasm of testis	M	5.3	5.4	5.1	6.0	5.8	6.0	6.3	6.9	6.8	6.6
C63	Malignant neoplasm of other and unspecified male genital organs	M	0.2	0.3	0.1	0.3	0.2	0.4	0.2	0.2	0.2	0.2
C64	Malignant neoplasm of kidney, except renal pelvis	M F	9.0 4.3	9.3 4.3	9.8 4.6	9.6 4.6	9.6 4.9	9.9 4.9	10.2 4.9	9.8 5.1	10.1 5.0	10.0 5.0
C65	Malignant neoplasm of renal pelvis	M F	0.5 0.2	0.5 0.2	0.5 0.3	0.5 0.3	0.5 0.3	0.6 0.4	0.6 0.3	0.6 0.3	0.7 0.4	0.7 0.3
C66	Malignant neoplasm of ureter	M F	0.5 0.2	0.5 0.2	0.4 0.2	0.5 0.2	0.4 0.2	0.4 0.2	0.4 0.2	0.5 0.2	0.6 0.3	0.6 0.2
C67	Malignant neoplasm of bladder	M F	30.5 8.6	30.6 8.6	30.0 7.9	30.5 8.4	28.4 7.8	27.2 8.0	27.3 7.7	26.5 7.8	23.1 6.5	21.8 6.1
C68	Malignant neoplasm of other and unspecified urinary organs	M F	0.3 0.1	0.3 0.1	0.3 0.1	0.3 0.1	0.3 0.1	1.0 0.3	0.2 0.1	0.2 0.1	0.3 0.1	0.3 0.1
C69	Malignant neoplasm of eye and adnexa	M F	1.0 0.8	0.9 0.7	0.8 0.6	0.9 0.8	0.7 0.6	0.9 0.7	0.7 0.5	0.6 0.5	0.8 0.6	0.7 0.5
C70	Malignant neoplasm of meninges	M F	0.1 0.1	0.1 0.0	0.1 0.1	0.1 0.2	0.1 0.1	0.1 0.1	0.1 0.1	0.1 0.1	0.1 0.1	0.1 0.1
C71	Malignant neoplasm of brain	M F	7.9 5.4	7.6 5.2	7.6 5.1	7.8 5.4	7.7 5.3	8.3 5.3	7.8 5.4	8.0 5.0	8.2 5.5	7.9 5.1
C72	Malignant neoplasm of spinal cord, cranial nerves and other parts of central nervous system	M F	0.2 0.1	0.2 0.2	0.2 0.2	0.3 0.2	0.3 0.2	0.3 0.3	0.2 0.2	0.2 0.2	0.2 0.3	0.2 0.2
C73	Malignant neoplasm of thyroid gland	M F	0.9 2.4	1.0 2.3	1.0 2.7	1.0 2.4	1.1 2.4	1.1 2.5	1.3 2.7	1.2 2.7	1.2 3.0	1.2 3.1

* Using the European standard population

Table 10 Directly age standardised* rates - *continued* England

ICD (10th Revision) number	Site description		1992	1993	1994	1995	1996	1997	1998	1999	2000	2001
C74	Malignant neoplasm of adrenal gland	M F	0.3 0.2	0.4 0.3	0.3 0.3	0.3 0.3	0.3 0.3	0.4 0.3	0.3 0.3	0.3 0.3	0.3 0.3	0.3 0.4
C75	Malignant neoplasm of other endocrine glands and related structures	M F	0.3 0.2	0.2 0.1	0.2 0.1	0.2 0.1	0.2 0.1	0.1 0.1	0.2 0.1	0.2 0.1	0.2 0.1	0.2 0.1
C76	Malignant neoplasm of other and ill-defined sites	M F	0.4 0.5	0.4 0.5	0.6 0.7	0.8 0.8	0.7 0.7	0.7 0.8	0.7 0.8	0.9 0.9	0.9 0.9	0.7 0.8
C77	Secondary and unspecified malignant neoplasm of lymph nodes	M F	0.9 0.7	1.0 0.9	1.3 1.0	1.0 0.9	1.7 1.1	1.7 1.2	1.2 0.8	1.4 0.8	1.3 0.9	1.3 0.9
C78	Secondary malignant neoplasm of respiratory and digestive organs	M F	6.5 4.9	6.9 5.3	7.1 5.6	7.1 5.3	6.7 5.3	6.8 5.3	6.7 5.1	6.9 5.2	6.6 4.8	6.6 5.5
C79	Secondary malignant neoplasm of other sites	M F	3.1 2.5	3.3 2.5	3.5 2.5	3.2 2.4	3.3 2.4	3.1 2.5	3.0 2.3	2.9 2.1	2.8 2.2	3.1 2.4
C80	Malignant neoplasm without specification of site	M F	11.5 8.4	11.6 8.4	11.0 8.2	11.0 8.7	11.7 8.7	11.7 9.1	11.2 8.2	10.3 8.4	8.6 7.5	7.9 7.2
C81	Hodgkin's disease	M F	2.8 1.8	2.7 1.8	2.5 1.9	2.6 1.8	2.5 1.8	2.6 1.8	2.8 2.0	2.7 1.9	3.0 2.0	2.7 1.9
C82-C85	Non-Hodgkin's lymphoma	M F	13.3 9.2	13.4 9.1	14.2 9.7	13.8 9.3	13.8 9.3	14.5 9.9	14.8 10.5	15.1 10.8	15.3 10.9	15.4 10.9
C88	Malignant immunoproliferative diseases	M F	0.0 0.0	0.1 0.0	0.1 0.0	0.4 0.2	0.3 0.1	0.4 0.2	0.5 0.2	0.5 0.3	0.4 0.2	0.5 0.2
C90	Multiple myeloma and malignant plasma cell neoplasms	M F	5.4 3.4	5.3 3.5	5.1 3.6	5.3 4.0	5.2 3.5	5.2 3.6	5.8 3.8	5.5 3.8	5.7 4.0	5.4 3.5
C91-C95	All leukaemias	M F	10.6 6.5	10.9 6.6	10.9 6.9	12.4 7.3	11.2 7.0	11.5 7.3	11.7 7.3	11.4 7.3	12.2 7.0	11.6 7.0
C91	Lymphoid leukaemia	M F	4.9 2.6	5.4 2.9	5.3 3.1	6.4 3.4	6.2 3.3	5.8 3.1	6.0 3.3	6.0 3.3	6.4 3.3	6.1 3.4
C92	Myeloid leukaemia	M F	4.9 3.4	4.8 3.3	5.0 3.4	5.3 3.6	4.5 3.3	5.2 3.8	5.0 3.6	4.8 3.6	5.1 3.3	5.0 3.3
C93	Monocytic leukaemia	M F	0.2 0.1	0.1 0.1	0.1 0.0	0.1 0.1	0.1 0.1	0.1 0.1	0.1 0.1	0.1 0.1	0.2 0.1	0.2 0.1
C94	Other leukaemias of specified cell type	M F	0.1 0.0	0.1 0.1	0.0 0.0	0.1 0.0	0.1 0.0	0.1 0.0	0.1 0.0	0.1 0.0	0.1 0.0	0.1 0.0
C95	Leukaemia of unspecified cell type	M F	0.6 0.3	0.5 0.3	0.4 0.3	0.4 0.2	0.4 0.2	0.4 0.3	0.4 0.3	0.4 0.3	0.4 0.2	0.3 0.2
C96	Other and unspecified malignant neoplasms of lymphoid, haematopoietic and related tissue	M F	0.2 0.1	0.2 0.2	0.1 0.1	0.0 0.1	0.2 0.2	0.4 0.2	0.1 0.0	0.1 0.0	0.0 0.0	0.1 0.0
D05	Carcinoma in situ of breast	F	7.0	6.6	6.6	7.2	7.5	8.7	9.5	10.5	11.2	11.6
D06	Carcinoma in situ of cervix uteri	F	71.6	69.3	74.5	79.3	81.9	80.2	87.9	87.4	82.7	79.2

* Using the European standard population

Appendix 1 Guidance notes and definitions

1   DATA

Cancer registrations

For the purposes of the national cancer registration scheme the term 'cancer' includes all malignant neoplasms and the reticuloses, that is conditions listed under site code numbers C00 to C97 of the Tenth Revision of the International Statistical Classification of Diseases and Related Health Problems[1]. In addition, all carcinoma in situ and neoplasms of uncertain behaviour are registered. Benign neoplasms and neoplasms of unspecified nature of bladder and brain, including the pineal and pituitary glands, are also registered, together with hydatidiform mole.

It should be noted that some cancer registries are not always able to collect complete information about benign, uncertain and unspecified neoplasms and therefore these registration rates are almost certainly underestimates of the true incidence. In particular, this should be noted when interpreting regional differences.

Quality of cancer registration data

A brief history of cancer registration in England and Wales is given above (pages 4-10). The essential features of the current system have remained unchanged for over 30 years. The main flows of information to and from the regional registries and ONS, including the National Health Service Central Register (NHSCR), are illustrated in Figure A on page 5. Some aspects of the system which are relevant to the interpretation of the data have been discussed in considerable detail by Swerdlow[2]. These and others including geographic coverage; methods of data collection; ascertainment (or completeness of registration); completeness of recording of data items; validity; accuracy; late registrations, deletions and amendments; duplicate and multiple registrations; registrations from information on death certificates; clinical and pathological definitions and diagnoses; changes in coding systems; completeness of flagging at NHSCR; changes in definition of resident population; and error, are discussed below.

Over the years, changes have occurred to the number of registries and to their **geographic coverage**. In 1950 there were 74 centres registering cancer in England and Wales, but the system was progressively simplified and by 1958 ten regions were covered by regional cancer registries; full coverage of England and Wales (but not 100% ascertainment of cases - see below) was achieved in 1962.

Some registries covered more than one RHA: the Thames Registry was formed in 1985 with the merger of the North West, North East and South Thames registries (the last of these covered both the South West and South East Thames RHAs). Wessex was separated from the South Thames registry in 1973; this coincided with a change in the method of data collection and a substantial increase in numbers of registrations for some parts of the Wessex region. Following reorganisations at the regional level in the NHS in 1996, the former South Western and Wessex RHAs are now covered by the South and West Cancer Intelligence Service based in Bristol and Winchester. The former Yorkshire RHA and part of the former Northern RHA are now covered by the Northern and Yorkshire Cancer Registry and Information Service based in Leeds (the remainder of the former Northern RHA, South Cumbria, is now covered by the North Western Registry). Further reorganisations at the regional level in the NHS occurred in 1999 and 2001, but no corresponding major changes have been made to the areas covered by the cancer registries. Some registries received reports from several centres in their areas - at various times five regional centres existed in Trent, two in South Western, and three in East Anglian.

The independent cancer registries differ considerably in their **methods of data collection**; some employ peripatetic clerks, others use hospital record staff to extract data for the registry, and several rely heavily on other organisations' computer systems including those in hospitals and pathology laboratories. The registries probably also differ in the level of **ascertainment** of their data (that is the degree to which reportable incident cases of cancer in the population are actually recorded in the registry) but the best are known to have very high levels. Direct measures are only available from occasional special studies[3,4]. That by Hawkins and Swerdlow[3] estimated that the under-ascertainment of registration of childhood cancers by the regional registries was just under 5%; under-ascertainment may be greater for adults, for whom registration and record linkage (in the registries and at NHSCR) may be more difficult, than for children. General indications of ascertainment levels can be obtained from comparisons of the numbers of registrations and deaths in a period. The figures for deaths are those coded to a particular type of cancer as the underlying cause of death in residents of the same geographical area. Such mortality to incidence ratios by sex and site for 2001 are presented in Table 9. These ratios have several limitations, but there are variations between regions (and over time) which would be difficult to explain unless there were similar variations in ascertainment.

It may be difficult to interpret any apparent trends in cancer registrations because the registries are continually striving to increase their levels of ascertainment of cases. Any particularly large increases from year to year in the numbers of registrations for an individual registry are most likely to have arisen because of this. For example, the recorded incidence for residents in some parts of the Thames Regional Health Authorities was unusually high in 1992, and unusually low in 1993, as a result of a one-off exercise by the Thames Cancer Registry in 1993 to find further information for people with cancer mentioned on their death certificate[5].

Completeness is the extent to which all appropriate data items have been recorded in the registry database. Some data items are essential; if high proportions of such items are missing, this is an indicator of poor quality. For example, for cases that have been registered solely from the information on a death certificate (DCO) the incidence date is unknown and has to be taken as the date of death and the case may well be recorded against the wrong calendar year. A high DCO rate also implies under-ascertainment[6] because patients are being missed by the registry while they are alive and not all cancer patients die of their disease (in which case, cancer is not mentioned on the death certificate). Other quality indicators are the proportion of cases where the primary site is unknown, and the proportions where important information such as the age of the patient or their postcode, is missing. Tables giving the proportions of registrations by region that have zero survival (which include both DCO cases and patients who were known to have died on the day of diagnosis - true zero survival) are given in Appendix E1 of the *Cancer Trends* volume[7]: and tables giving the proportions of registrations by region with site unspecified are given in its Appendix E2.

The agreed procedures to be followed by the cancer registries and ONS when submitting and processing data

Figure 1A Number of newly diagnosed cases of cancer* by quality status†, as at July 2004, England, 1971-2001

Year	Total	Status 1	Status 2	Status 3	Status 3 as % of total
1971	143876	141401	2151	324	0.2
1972	146408	144226	1840	342	0.2
1973	151766	149490	1886	390	0.3
1974	156617	155497	619	501	0.3
1975	157009	155958	432	619	0.4
1976	157902	156278	869	755	0.5
1977	160816	159859	164	793	0.5
1978	160768	159848	161	759	0.5
1979	163824	162951	258	615	0.4
1980	169425	168514	300	611	0.4
1981	174143	171957	1423	763	0.4
1982	175130	172842	1534	754	0.4
1983	178514	175713	2010	791	0.4
1984	178570	174803	2811	956	0.5
1985	189393	187259	1312	822	0.4
1986	186097	183541	1637	919	0.5
1987	191339	188430	2092	817	0.4
1988	197419	194033	2407	979	0.5
1989	197580	193747	2777	1056	0.5
1990	198933	179726	18918	289	0.1
1991	202066	198257	3598	211	0.1
1992	210577	206237	3778	562	0.3
1993	208386	203555	4368	463	0.2
1994	212832	212036	372	424	0.2
1995	215374	214902	29	443	0.2
1996	214887	214483	28	376	0.2
1997	221796	221511	67	218	0.1
1998	221602	221345	36	221	0.1
1999	227602	226765	524	313	0.1
2000	226964	226843	17	104	0.0
2001	227756	227606	7	143	0.1

* All malignant neoplasms excluding non-melonoma skin cancer
† See text

are set out in the 'Registry/ONS Interface Document'[8]. When a registry's submission is loaded onto the database at ONS, a large number of **validity** checks are carried out. There are over 40 checks on individual data items. These include that dates are valid, or that an 'indicator' is either 0 or 1 (or '&' if not known). There are around 20 cross checks between data items. These include the consistency of dates, for example that the incidence date is not after the date of death, and that the cancer site and histology are compatible. These latter cross checks are based closely on those promulgated by the International Agency for Research on Cancer (IARC)[6] and used by them when verifying data for inclusion in *Cancer Incidence in Five Continents*[9]. Combinations of site and histology are checked against three lists:

(i) histology codes which will be accepted in combination with any site code;
(ii) histology codes which will only be accepted if the site code is in the appropriate group (of which there are over 50); and
(iii) histology codes which will not be accepted in combination with any of the sites in a group (of which there are two).

If a record passes all the checks and cross checks, it is given a quality status of 1. If a record fails any one of a small number of vital checks and cross checks, for example if the date of birth is invalid, thus making it impossible either to include the data in an output table in the ONS annual reference volume[5] or to flag the person concerned at the NHSCR, it is given a quality status of 3. If a record passes all the vital checks and cross checks but fails one or more other checks, it is given a quality status of 2, and along with records that have a quality status of 1, can be used in outputs and sent to the NHSCR for flagging. Information about all records which fail any of the validation checks is sent to the registries for them to investigate and submit corrections.

The national standards for cancer registries[10,11] require that when a registry's data for a particular year are complete, no more than 0.5% of records should have a quality status of 3. When OPCS redeveloped its cancer registration computer processing system in the early 1990s, all the previously submitted records were re-validated using the more stringent checks[8] incorporated in the new system. The quality status of all the records on the database at the National Cancer Intelligence Centre (NCIC) from 1971 up to 2001 is shown in Figure 1A. Over the past ten years, the proportion of records with serious errors has consistently been 0.2% or less.

As with completeness, the **accuracy** of the data (that is the proportion of cases recorded with a given characteristic that truly have the attribute) is only occasionally known directly from special studies. Various indirect measures, however, suggest that there is considerable variation between regions. A report of a project to audit the quality and comparability of cancer registration data in the UK, carried out under the aegis of the United Kingdom Association of Cancer Registries (see above) was published in 1995[12]. Variations among the registries were found in data quality for diagnostic factors, incidence date, stage of disease, treatment information, and use of death information. A study at the Merseyside and Cheshire Registry[13] also found that data quality within a registry varied by the age of the patient, the cancer site, and area of residence. However, a substantial audit of Scottish cancer registry data[14], in which information was re-abstracted from the available records, found that severe discrepancies had occurred in under 3% of cases. The review[12] concluded that although comparisons between the various published studies was difficult, cancer registry records were largely complete, accurate and reliable. The review found that the quality of cancer registry data depended heavily on the competence and experience of staff in the registry; on maintaining good relationships with clinicians, staff in health authorities, and scientists; and on the registry's active involvement in research.

The point in time at which ONS, in consultation with the cancer registries, decides to produce the tables for the reference volume is necessarily a compromise between two principal considerations - the need to minimise the delay between the relevant data year and the publication of the detailed results, and the requirement to obtain a very high level of completeness of the data and hence minimise the number of **late registrations**. The gap between the data year and production of tables has varied considerably; as a result there are currently varying proportions of additional cancer registrations held on the computer files at ONS compared with the numbers published in the corresponding reference volume, as shown in Figure 1B. Over the twenty nine year period the differences have averaged around

Figure 1B   Number of registrations (thousands) published in ARVs and currently (July 2004) on the NCIC database, England

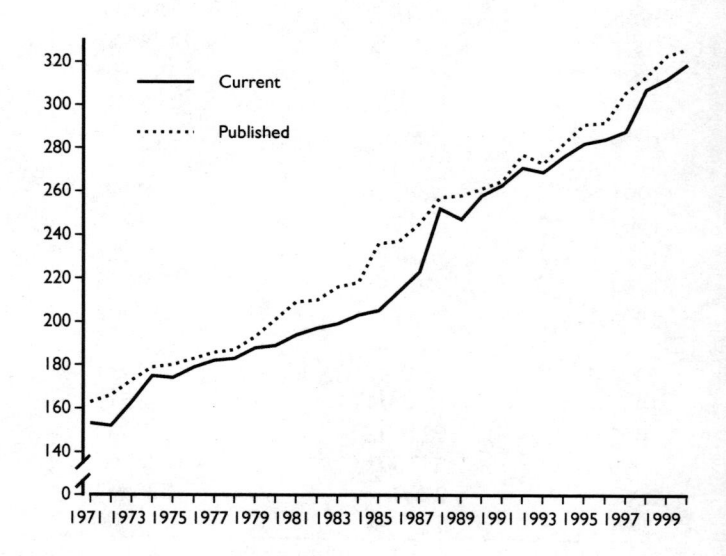

3% although the differences for 1985, 1986 and 1987 are larger as a result of the problems with the transmission of data between the Thames Registry and ONS[15]. The overall figures contain within them some substantial variations among the regions. For example, a problem at OPCS (as it was then) with the processing of one data tape for 1985 from the North Western registry resulted in a shortfall in the published figures of around two thousand registrations. Although this made a difference of less than 1 per cent to the total for England and Wales, it represented a shortfall of around 10 per cent for the North Western region. **Late deletions and amendments** to data are in general a much smaller problem than late new registrations.

A CD-ROM containing anonymised records of new cases of cancer - including all the 'late' registrations - for incidence years 1971 to 1992 has been produced by ONS[16]; the data are geographically coded to regional health authority level. Also included are anonymised records of deaths from cancer for 1971-1997; and the relevant mid-year population estimates to enable the calculation of incidence and mortality rates. The NCIC plans to update this CD-ROM with incidence data for 1991-1999 and cancer mortality data for 1991-2000.

While late registrations result in the figures published in the reference volume being too low, **duplicate registrations** can artificially inflate them. Such duplication may arise if a patient is resident in one area but treated in another; this is particularly so for those resident in North Wales and treated in Liverpool, and for those resident around London who are treated in central London. Duplications are prevented firstly by the cancer registries which hold alphabetic indexes of names and carry out computer searches; and secondly by the flagging at NHSCR, where if on flagging, a previous registration is found for the individual, the registrations are examined to see if they are duplicates or **true multiple primary** cancers. The rules for decisions on duplicates/multiples have changed over time, particularly for 1978 registrations which led to a 13 per cent decrease in registrations for Welsh residents. Currently, with the agreement of the cancer registries, all such cases are referred back to them by ONS, and decisions taken according to an agreed set of rules[8].

Since the early 1960s, copies of information from all death certificates mentioning cancer have been sent by ONS to the registry covering the area in which the death occurred. Any cancers registered solely from the information on the death certificates were not included in the published information prior to 1974, at which point an abrupt increase occurred. Registries use the death certificate information in different ways. For example, some check the data by reference to clinical notes or other local data sources, but others simply enter the death as a registration (with the year of death as the incidence year).

Inaccuracies and incompleteness may arise from **diagnostic practice**, and changes in it, although such errors and changes come from outside the cancer registration system and are not under its control. Misclassification of cancers is more likely to occur when there is no opportunity to obtain histological confirmation of disease, or if the tumour has a pre-malignant stage which can be confused with invasive carcinoma. Misclassification may also result from mistakes in the collection, abstraction or coding of information both before and after it reaches the registry. Also, **clinical and pathological** (and registry) **definitions of cancer** may change over time and between places, particularly for borderline malignant conditions.

Changes in **coding systems** may cause discontinuities in published data. For the national data held by ONS, for incidence years 1971 to 1978, site is coded to ICD8 and histology by the Manual of Tumor Nomenclature and Coding (MOTNAC) 1968 edition[17]; for incidence years 1979 to 1994, site is coded to ICD9 and histology to ICD-O[18]; and from incidence year 1995 onwards, site is coded to ICD10 and histology to ICD-O2[1]. Details of the effect of the changes between the ICD revisions on mortality statistics have been published[19]; these give an indication of their likely effect on cancer registrations. In addition, there have been some minor changes in ONS coding and classification rules[3]. Over time the submission of data from the registries to ONS on abstract cards was superseded by computer media (punched cards, magnetic tape and diskettes). Abstract cards were coded at ONS whereas magnetic tapes and diskettes were coded by the registry before being sent to ONS. Thus a change to magnetic tape (the last registry to do so was Oxford in 1985) may have been accompanied by changes in interpretation of coding.

In addition, the **completeness of flagging** of registrations by NHSCR is important for cohort studies. The proportion of cancer registrations received by ONS which were successfully linked to an NHSCR record was on average about 96 per cent from 1971 up to 1989. With the computerisation at NHSCR and improvements in data quality by the regional cancer registries, this has risen to over 99% for data for 1993 and subsequent years. The importance for any particular study of the records not traced will depend upon any biases by area, cancer site or other main factors of interest[20].

Rates of cancer incidence are dependent not only on the accuracy of the cancer registration data but also on that of the **population denominator data**. Recent censuses are believed to have been very accurate overall: under-enumeration in 1981 was estimated to be 0.5 per cent (240,000 people) and in 1991 to be 1.1 per cent (572,000 people), but this varied by age and by geographic area. Annual mid-year estimates of population, based on census data together with information on births, deaths and migration (see above) also appear to be very accurate on a national basis, although errors of several per cent have been found for some counties, districts and London boroughs. There may also be differences between the definitions of 'place of residence' used for cancer registrations and for population estimates. For the former, the address used is 'the usual place of residence as given by the patient', whereas the census definition is not so straightforward, particularly when a person lives at more than one address throughout the year[21]. This may lead to biases in analyses of data for small areas which include large numbers of students, armed forces or people living in institutions.

Although the census population figures for 2001 were overall some 1 million lower than the previously published population estimates, the differences were concentrated largely in the younger age groups, particularly for males. Cancer is a disease predominantly of older people, and checks on data for England and Wales have shown that in general the effects on overall cancer incidence rates of using populations for the 1990s that have been revised in the light of the results of the 2001 census, and subsequently, are very small.

Finally, in published data on the scale of the national cancer registration system it is almost inevitable that straightforward **errors** will occur, for example in the transcription and printing of tables. Corrections to known errors have been published.

Mortality data

Most deaths are certified by a medical practitioner. The death certificate is then usually taken to a registrar of births and deaths by a person known as an informant - usually a near relative of the deceased. In certain cases, deaths are referred to, and sometimes then investigated by, a coroner who sends information to the registrar of deaths which is used instead of that from the medical practitioner. In some cases, additional information from the coroner's certificate is forwarded to ONS by the registrar. Thus the information used in ONS mortality statistics may have come from one of four sources: the doctor, the informant, a coroner, or derived from one or other of the above (for example, the age of the dead person is derived from date of birth and date of death).

In the early 1990s, OPCS redeveloped its deaths registrations computer processing system. The main changes affecting the data included the progressive computerisation of local offices of registrars of births and deaths, and the automation of cause of death coding.

A full set of notes and definitions for mortality data has been published by ONS[22]. This includes: base populations; occurrences and registrations; areal coverage; death rates and standardisation; certification of cause of death; coding the underlying cause of death; analysis of conditions mentioned on the death certificate; amended cause of death; accelerated registrations; legislation on registration of deaths and the processing, reporting and analysis of mortality data; and historical changes in mortality data including the introduction of the Ninth Revision of the International Classification of Diseases[18] in 1979, industrial action taken by registration officers in 1981-82, and the amendment by OPCS in 1984 of WHO Rule 3 (one of the rules used to select the underlying cause of death).

Further information is provided in reference 22 about the redevelopment of the deaths computer processing system, the use of 'medical enquiries' to the certifier of death for further information in order to assign a more definite code, and the use of WHO Rule 3. There is also advice on using cause of death from 1993 onwards.

The main change in introducing automated cause of death coding was in the interpretation of WHO Rule 3. The death certificate is set out in two parts; part I gives the condition or sequence of conditions leading to death, while part II gives details of any associated conditions. Rule 3 states that 'if the condition selected by the General rules or Rules 1 and 2 can be considered a direct sequel of another reported condition, whether in part I or part II, select this primary condition'[18]. The interpretation of Rule 3 was broadened by OPCS in 1984 so that certain conditions which were often terminal, such as bronchopneumonia or pulmonary embolism, could be considered a direct sequel of any more specific condition reported. The more specific condition would then be regarded as the underlying cause. This change in interpretation meant that the numbers of deaths from certain conditions such as pneumonia fell suddenly in 1984, while deaths from conditions often mentioned in part II of the certificate rose[23]. The change in 1993 was a move back to the internationally accepted interpretation of Rule 3 operating in England and Wales before 1984.

Information on the effects of moving back to this earlier interpretation of Rule 3 have been published[24,25]. The expected effects were based on the assumption that any allowance for them was the same in 1993 as it was in 1984 (which is unlikely to be exactly true). But the effects of the change appear to be generally in the opposite direction to those of 1984 and of a similar magnitude[22].

Since January 2001, cause of death has been coded to ICD10[1]. Under ICD10, the interpretation of WHO Rule 3 is different from that in ICD9,[18] but similar to that adopted by OPCS for deaths in 1984-1992 (see above). In order to quantify the effects of this and other differences between ICD9 and ICD10, ONS carried out a bridge coding study: all deaths registered in 1999 were independently coded to both ICD9 and ICD10, and the causes compared using internationally agreed groups of equivalent codes. The full results can be found in the Report 'Results of the ICD bridge coding study, England and Wales, 1999' in *Health Statistics Quarterly* 14.[26] The numbers of deaths coded to "malignant neoplasms" in ICD10 were higher than in ICD9 by around three per cent for males and two per cent for females.

Quality of mortality data

As explained above, mortality statistics in England and Wales are derived from the registration of deaths certified by a doctor or coroner. The data pass through a number of processes before becoming usable for analysis. These processes are complex, and involve a wide range of people, organisations and computer systems. The scope for error is correspondingly wide. ONS aims to produce mortality statistics with the highest achievable quality given the available resources.

The quality checks and validations carried out at the various stages in the creation of mortality statistics are described in detail in reference 22. These include: writing the medical certificate of death; registration of the death; entry of data in the computer system used by registrars of births and deaths; other checks made by the registration service; receipt of death registration data at ONS; validation processes; routine checks by ONS; the automated cause coding system; checks before and after extraction of data for analysis; checks on routine outputs; and analysis of ill-defined causes of death.

Advantages and disadvantages of incidence and mortality data

In 1981, Doll and Peto[27] compared the quality and utility of incidence and mortality data in the USA. The incidence data came from two 'one off' national cancer surveys in 1947/48 and 1969-71, and from continuous collection up to 1977 by the Surveillance, Epidemiology and End Results (SEER) cancer registries (which operated in various cities and states and in total covered about 10% of the US population). They showed that mortality data were largely reliable and stable over time. But examples for a few major sites such as breast (in females) and prostate indicated that there were discrepancies with incidence that were too large to be explained without there being serious upward biases in the trends in cancer registration data, and that mortality data were generally more trustworthy.

These conclusions do not apply to cancer registration data in the UK. As noted above, a recent review of the quality of UK cancer registry data[12] concluded that results were largely complete, accurate and reliable. The data on cancer registration 'quality indicators' - mortality to incidence ratios, zero survival cases, and unspecified site - demonstrate that although there is some variability within England and Wales, the overall ascertainment and reliability is good. And the trends in incidence and mortality illustrated for the major cancer sites in Chapter 2 of the *Cancer Trends* volume[7] clearly confirm that, although there may have been some under registration, particularly for lung and stomach cancer, in the early 1970s, from the late 1970s onwards the trends in incidence are consistent with those for mortality and the recorded improvements in survival[28,29].

Mortality data are generally more timely than incidence (the current gap is two years - the latest mortality data[31] are for 2003[30], while incidence data are available up to 2001). This is largely because there is a statutory requirement to register a death within five days, and for the large majority of deaths there is only one source document. As explained above, cancer registration is not statutory and collating information from the necessary wide variety of sources is time consuming, and ONS cannot produce final results for England and Wales until data have been received from all registries. But trends in mortality give only a delayed

Figure 1C Advantages and disadvantages of incidence and mortality data

Incidence	Mortality
Advantages • high quality coding • both cancer site and histology • very low proportion site unspecified • incidence date known (except for small proportion registered solely from a death certificate)	**Disadvantages** • diagnostic accuracy less certain than for incidence • site only, no histology • around 10% site unspecified • deaths in any one year result from cases diagnosed over a long previous period
Disadvantages • may not be complete • may not be sufficiently timely • national coverage not achieved until 1962; evidence of under-ascertainment in the early 1970s	**Advantages** • virtually 100% complete • timely (within months of the end of a data year) • very long time series (if not affected by ICD or other coding changes[19])

indication of trends in new cases, because for cancers with moderate or good survival, those dying in any one year may have been diagnosed and treated many years earlier. Even in the 1970s, five year survival from many of the major cancers, for example breast (in females), cervix, larynx, melanoma of skin, testis and uterus, was in the range 50-70% and since then there have been notable improvements in survival for almost all except the highly fatal cancers (lung, oesophagus, pancreas)[28,29]. This has made incidence data increasingly more important for early monitoring of trends, and for assessment of major public health interventions such as breast and cervical screening[32-35].

Mortality data never were free from bias or criticism[36]. Death is not always correctly certified, or the underlying cause correctly coded, even for cancer. Many studies have shown wide variability in certification and coding, particularly between countries[37-48]. Although the mortality data are virtually 100% complete, while cancer registration data may not be, around 10% of deaths in England and Wales are coded to 'site unspecified'[22], whereas the corresponding proportion for incidence data is only 3%. These and other advantages and disadvantages of incidence and mortality data are summarised in Figure 1C.

Cancer mortality trends are therefore an imperfect and fuzzy indicator of trends in the efficacy of treatment - they reflect earlier trends in both incidence and survival and cannot be interpreted sensibly without them. Incidence and survival trends from the national cancer registry, based on data from the regional cancer registries, provide additional insight into the complex problems of cancer control. None of these indicators is perfect, and none is adequate on its own[49].

Populations

The population figures for 2001 used to calculate incidence rates given in this volume are the published ONS mid-year estimates of the population resident in England, revised as a consequence of the provisional results from the Manchester matching exercise. The latest population estimates, incorporating the results from the local authority studies, published on 9 September 2004 were not available when this volume was prepared. The mid-1990 estimates and those for later years are not directly comparable with those produced for years before 1981: residents who were outside Great Britain on census night are now included whereas overseas visitors to Great Britain are now excluded.

Table 2 contains the population estimates for England by sex and age for 2001. Users requiring further information on these estimates should contact the Population Estimates Unit at: Office for National Statistics, Segensworth Road, Titchfield, Fareham, Hants, PO15 5RR.

Occasional Paper No. 37 describes methods used by ONS to produce annual mid-year estimates of the population of local and health authority areas in England and Wales. It includes historical background and methods used in the 1980s. Details are given of the components of change (births, deaths and migration), and of methods used to estimate some special groups in the population, such as students and armed forces. Methods for re-basing the estimates for the 1990s, incorporating the results of the 1991 Census, are also included. The paper is available, price £4.00, from Customer Enquiry Centre at: Office for National Statistics, Government Buildings, Cardiff Road, Newport, South Wales, NP10 8XG.

Government offices for the regions (GORs)

Regional incidence data in this annual reference volume are presented by the patient's government office for the region of usual residence.

Some cancer registry publications present statistics based on the number of patients treated in the cancer registry area. Statistics in some cancer registry reports may therefore differ from the analyses by region of residence given in this volume.

2 METHODS

Age standardised rates

The incidence of cancer varies greatly with age. Differences in the age structure of populations between geographical areas or over time therefore need to be controlled to give unbiased comparisons of incidence. This can be achieved through either direct or indirect standardisation[50].

(i) Direct standardisation: Age and sex specific rates in each group in the populations to be compared are multiplied by the corresponding number of people in a 'standard' population, usually the World or (here) European standards - see Appendix F of the *Cancer Trends* volume[7], and then summed to give an overall rate per 100,000 population.

Thus the directly standardised incidence rate using the European standard population is given by

$$I(ASR/E) = \left\{ \sum_k i_k P_k \right\} / \sum_k P_k$$

where i_k = observed incidence rate in age group k
  k = 1, ... , 19 and the 19 age groups are 0, 1-4, 5-9, ... , 80-84, and 85 and over
  P_k = standard population in age group k

Such directly standardised rates are presented in Table 10 which gives time series for 1992 to 2001.

(ii) Indirect standardisation: Here, one set of age and sex specific rates (here those for England as a whole) is taken as the standard. These rates are then applied to each of several index populations of known age structure to show how many registrations would have been expected in these index populations had they, at each age, experienced the cancer incidence of the standard population. The 'expected' incidence so found is then compared with the observed, their ratio being multiplied by 100 to give an index, called the standardised registration ratio (SRR), in which 100 is the value for the standard population. Calculations are based on nineteen age groups (those used in Table 1).

The use of the SRR enables data for a particular site and sex to be presented as a single index figure relative to a defined standard or baseline. If the incidence patterns in the various age groups are different in the two populations or time periods, however, SRRs are an unreliable guide to comparison, and age-specific rates should be examined.

Table 6 shows the SRRs in GORs of residence for 2001. For each cancer, the registration rates in England are taken as standards (with the sexes considered separately). For example, the SRR for cancer of the stomach in the East Midlands GOR was calculated as:

$$SRR = 100 \times \frac{\text{No. of registrations of cancer of the stomach in East Midlands GOR}}{\sum_{\text{Age group}} \left[\begin{array}{l} \text{Population in each age group, East} \\ \text{Midlands GOR} \times \text{registration rate for} \\ \text{cancer of the stomach for that age, England} \end{array} \right]}$$

Cumulative lifetime risk

The risk of a person developing cancer during their lifetime is obtained by applying sex- and age-specific incidence rates to the person years at risk derived from the numbers of survivors from a hypothetical cohort based on an England life table. It gives the percent of the cohort that would develop cancer should the current age and sex specific rates be experienced throughout the lifetime of the cohort[51]. It can also be expressed as the odds of developing the disease during a person's lifetime.

Survival

ONS registrations since 1971 have been linked at the NHSCR to the death records (as already described); national survival tables have been published in *Cancer Survival Trends in England and Wales, 1971-1995: deprivation and NHS region*[28], and extended in *Cancer Survival in England and Wales, 1991-98*[29], *Cancer Survival 1992-1999*[52]; *Cancer Survival, England, 1993-2000*[53]; *Cancer Survival, England and Wales 1991-2001*[54]; and *Trends and socioeconomic inequalities in cancer survival in England and Wales up to 2001*[55].

The results of the first EUROCARE cancer survival study, which covered 30 cancer registries in 12 European countries, including England and Scotland, were published[56] in 1995. Six cancer registries in England participated; these were geographically spread around the country and covered almost half the population. Cancer registration data up to 1985 were included.

Results from the second EUROCARE study which covered 45 cancer registries in 17 countries, also including England and Scotland, have also been published[57, 58]. Seven cancer registries in England participated. Cancer registration data up to 1989 were included.

Some results from the third EUROCARE study which covered 56 cancer registries in 22 countries, including eight English registries and the registries in Wales and Scotland, were released at the European Cancer Conference (ECCO 12) in September 2003; full results were published in the journal *Annals of Oncology*[59]. Cancer registration data up to 1994 were included in the study.

Symbols and conventions used

-	nil
..	not available
:	not appropriate
nos	not otherwise specified
nec	not elsewhere classified

Further information

As noted above, individual anonymised records of new cases of cancer diagnosed from 1971 to 1992, together with individual anonymised records of deaths from cancer from 1971 to 1997, have been made available on a CD-ROM,[16] which can be purchased from ONS.

Special tabulations involving data not on the CD-ROM are available to order (subject to confidentiality thresholds) and on repayment. Such requests or enquiries should be made to:

National Cancer Intelligence Centre
Office for National Statistics
B7/04
1 Drummond Gate
London SW1V 2QQ

References

1. World Health Organisation. *International Statistical Classification of Diseases and Related Health Problems - Tenth Revision*. Geneva: WHO, 1992.
2. Swerdlow AJ. Cancer registration in England and Wales: Some aspects relevant to interpretation of the data. *Journal of the Royal Statistical Society Series A* 1986; **149**: 146-160.
3. Hawkins MM, Swerdlow AJ. Completeness of cancer and death follow-up obtained through the National Health Service Central Register for England and Wales. *British Journal of Cancer* 1992; **66**: 408-413.
4. Villard-Mackintosh L, Coleman MP, Vessey MP. The completeness of cancer registration in England: an assessment from Oxford FPA study. *British Journal of Cancer* 1988; **58**: 507-511.
5. Office for National Statistics. *Cancer statistics - registrations, England and Wales, 1993*. Series MB1 no.26. London: The Stationery Office, 1999.
6. Parkin DM, Chen VW, Ferlay J, Galceran J, Storm HH, Whelan SL. *Comparability and Quality Control in Cancer Registration*. IARC Technical Report No.19. Lyons: International Agency for Research on Cancer, 1994.
7. Quinn M J, Babb P J, Brock A, Kirby E A, Jones J. *Cancer Trends in England and Wales, 1950-1999*. Studies on Medical and Population Subjects No.66. London: The Stationery Office, 2001.
8. Office of Population Censuses and Surveys. *Registry/ONS Interface Document. National Cancer Registration System, England and Wales*. London: OPCS, 1994 (subsequently revised).
9. Parkin DM, Whelan SL, Ferlay J, Teppo L and Thomas DB, (eds). *Cancer Incidence in Five Continents, Vol. VIII*. IARC Scientific Publications No.155. Lyons: International Agency for Research on Cancer, 2003.
10. NHS Executive. *Core contract for purchasing Cancer Registration*. EL(96)7. London: NHS Executive, 1996. Winyard G. *EL(96)7: Core contract for purchasing cancer registration* (letter). Leeds: NHS Executive, 1998.
11. Department of Health. *Cancer Registry Standards for England, v2.1*. London: DH, 2001.
12. Huggett C. *Review of the Quality and Comparability of Data held by Regional Cancer Registries*. Bristol: Bristol Cancer Epidemiology Unit incorporating the South West Cancer Registry, 1995.
13. Seddon DJ, Williams EMI. Data quality in population based cancer registration: an assessment of the Merseyside and Cheshire Cancer Registry. *British Journal of Cancer* 1997; **76**: 667-674.
14. Brewster D, Crichton J, Muir C. How accurate are Scottish cancer registration data? *British Journal of Cancer* 1994; **70**: 954-959.
15. Office of Population Censuses and Surveys. *Cancer statistics – registrations, England and Wales, 1988*. Series MB1 no.21. London: HMSO, 1994.
16. Quinn MJ, Babb PJ, Jones J, Baker A, Ault C. *Cancer 1971-1997. Registrations of cancer cases and deaths in England and Wales by sex, age, year, health region and type of cancer* (CD-ROM). London: Office for National Statistics, 1999.
17. American Cancer Society. *Manual of tumor nomenclature and coding (MOTNAC)*. Washington DC: American Cancer Society, 1951.
18. World Health Organisation. *International Classification of Diseases - Ninth Revision*. Geneva: WHO, 1977.
19. Office of Population Censuses and Surveys. *Mortality statistics - comparison of 8th and 9th Revision of the International Classification of Diseases*. Series DH1 no.10. London: HMSO, 1983.
20. Quinn MJ. Progress on flagging cancers at NHSCR. *The Researcher* 2000; **14**: 4-5.
21. Office of Population Censuses and Surveys and General Register Office (Scotland). *1991 Census: Definitions, Great Britain*. London: HMSO, 1992.
22. Office for National Statistics. *Mortality statistics 1998: cause, England and Wales*. Series DH2 no.25. London: The Stationery Office, 1999.
23. Office of Population Censuses and Surveys. *Mortality statistics 1984: cause, England and Wales*. Series DH2 no.11. London: HMSO, 1985.
24. Office for National Statistics. *Mortality statistics 1993 (revised) and 1994: cause, England and Wales*. Series DH2 no.21. London: The Stationery Office, 1996.
25. Rooney C, Devis T. Mortality trends by cause of death in England and Wales 1980-94: the impact of introducing automated cause coding and related changes in 1993. *Population Trends* 1996; **86**: 29-35.
26. Office for National Statistics. Report: Results of the ICD10 bridge coding study, England and Wales, 1999. *Health Statistics Quarterly* 2002; **14**: 75-83.
27. Doll R, Peto R. *The Causes of Cancer*. Oxford: Oxford University Press, 1981.
28. Coleman MP, Babb P, Damiecki P, Grosclaude P, Honjo S, Jones J, Knerer G, Pitard A, Quinn MJ, Sloggett A, De Stavola B. *Cancer Survival Trends in England and Wales, 1971-1995: deprivation and NHS Region*. Studies in Medical and Population Subjects No. 61. London: The Stationery Office, 1999.
29. Coleman MP, Babb PJ, Harris S, Quinn MJ, Sloggett A, De Stavola BL. Report: Cancer survival in England and Wales, 1991-98. *Health Statistics Quarterly* 2000; **6**: 71-80.
30. Office for National Statistics. Report: Death registrations in England and Wales, 2003: causes. *Health Statistics Quarterly* 2004; **22**: 55-62.
31. Office for National Statistics. *Mortality Statistics 2002: England and Wales*. Series DH2 no.29. London: ONS, 2003.

32. Quinn MJ, Allen EJ, on behalf of the United Kingdom Association of Cancer Registries. Changes in incidence of and mortality from breast cancer in England and Wales since introduction of screening. *British Medical Journal* 1995; **311**: 1391-1395.
33. Blanks RG, Moss SM, McGahan CE, Quinn MJ, Babb PJ. Effect of NHS breast screening programme on mortality from breast cancer in England and Wales, 1990-8: comparison of observed with predicted mortality. *British Medical Journal* 2000; **321**: 665-669.
34. Quinn MJ, Babb PJ, Jones J, Allen E, on behalf of the United Kingdom Association of Cancer Registries. The effect of screening on the incidence of and mortality from cancer of the cervix in England: evaluation based on routinely collected statistics. *British Medical Journal* 1999; **318**: 904-908.
35. Sasieni P, Adams J. Effect of screening on cervical cancer mortality in England and Wales: analysis of trends with an age-cohort model. *British Medical Journal* 1999; **318**: 1244-1245.
36. Defoe D. *A journal of the plague year*. London, 1722.
37. Heasman MA, Lipworth L. *Accuracy of certification of cause of death*. Studies in Medical and Population Subjects no.20. London: HMSO, 1966.
38. Alderson MR, Meade TW. Accuracy of diagnosis on death certificates compared with that in hospital records. *British Journal of Preventive and Social Medicine* 1967; **21**: 22-29.
39. Grulich AE, Swerdlow AJ, dos Santos Silva I, Beral V. Is the apparent rise in cancer mortality in the elderly real? Analysis of changes in certification and coding of cause of death in England and Wales, 1970-1990. *International Journal of Cancer* 1995; **63**: 164-168.
40. Percy CL, Muir CS. The international comparability of cancer mortality data: results of an international death certificate study. *American Journal of Epidemiology* 1989; **129**: 934-946.
41. Ashworth TG. Inadequacy of death certification: proposal for change. *Journal of Clinical Patholology* 1991; **44**: 265-268.
42. Percy CL, Dolman AB. Comparison of the coding of death certificates related to cancer in seven countries. *Public Health Reports* 1978; **93**: 335-350.
43. Percy CL, Stanek E, Gloeckler Ries LA. Accuracy of cancer death certificates and its effect on cancer mortality statistics. *American Journal of Public Health* 1981; **71**: 242-250.
44. Percy CL, Miller BA, Gloeckler Ries LA. Effect of changes in cancer classification and the accuracy of cancer death certificates on trends in cancer mortality. *Annals of the New York Academy of Sciences* 1990; **609**: 87-97.
45. Hoel DG, Ron E, Carter R, Mabuchi K. Influence of death certificate errors on cancer mortality trends. *Journal of the National Cancer Institute* 1993; **85**: 1063-1068.
46. Lindahl BI, Johansson LA. Multiple cause-of-death data as a tool for detecting artificial trends in the underlying cause statistics: a methodological study. *Scandinavian Journal of Social Medicine* 1994; **22**: 145-158.
47. Garne JP, Aspegren K, Balldin G. Breast cancer as cause of death – a study over the validity of the officially registered cause of death in 2631 breast cancer patients dying in Malmö, Sweden 1964-1992. *Acta Oncologica* 1996; **35**: 671-675.
48. Jablon S, Thompson D, McConney M, Mabuchi K. Accuracy of cause-of-death certification in Hiroshima and Nagasaki, Japan. *Annals of the New York Academy of Sciences* 1990; **609**: 100-109.
49. Coleman MP, Babb PJ, Stockton D, Forman D, Møller H. Trends in breast cancer incidence, survival and mortality in England and Wales. *Lancet* 2000; **356**: 590-591 (letter).
50. dos Santos Silva I. *Cancer Epidemiology: Principles and Methods*. Lyons: International Agency for Research on Cancer, 1999.
51. Schouten LJ, Straatman H, Kiemeney LALM, Verbeek ALM. Cancer incidence: life table risk versus cumulative risk. *Journal of Epidemiology and Community Health* 1994; **48**: 596-600.
52. Office for National Statistics. *Cancer Survival 1992-1999*. London: ONS, 2001.
53. Office for National Statistics. *Cancer survival, England, 1993-2000*. London: ONS, 2002.
54. Office for National Statistics. *Cancer survival, England and Wales, 1991-2001*. London: ONS, 2003.
55. Coleman MP, Rachet B, Woods L, Mitry E, Riga M, Cooper N, Quinn MJ, Brenner H and Estève J. Trends and socioeconomic inequalities in cancer survival in England and Wales up to 2001. *British Journal of Cancer* 2004; **90**: 1367-1313.
56. Berrino F, Sant M, Verdechia A, Capocaccia R, Hakulinen T, Estève J (eds). *Survival of cancer patients in Europe. The EUROCARE Study*. Lyons: International Agency for Research on Cancer, IARC Scientific Publication No.132, 1995.
57. Coebergh JWW, Sant M, Berrino F, Verdecchia A (eds). *Survival of Adult Cancer Patients diagnosed from 1978-1989: The EUROCARE II Study*. European Journal of Cancer 1998, **34**, 2137-2278.
58. Berrino F, Sant M, Verdechia A, Capocaccia R, Hakulinen T, Estève J (eds). *Survival of cancer patients in Europe during 1985-1989. EUROCARE II*. Lyons: International Agency for Research on Cancer, IARC Scientific Publication No. 151, 1999.
59. Micheli A, Baili P, Quinn MJ, Mugno E, Capocaccia R, Groscloude P and the EUROCARE working group. Life expectancy and cancer survival in EUROCARE-3 cancer registry areas. *Annals of Onology* 2003; **14** (Supp 15): v28-v40.

Appendix 2 Maps and contact addresses

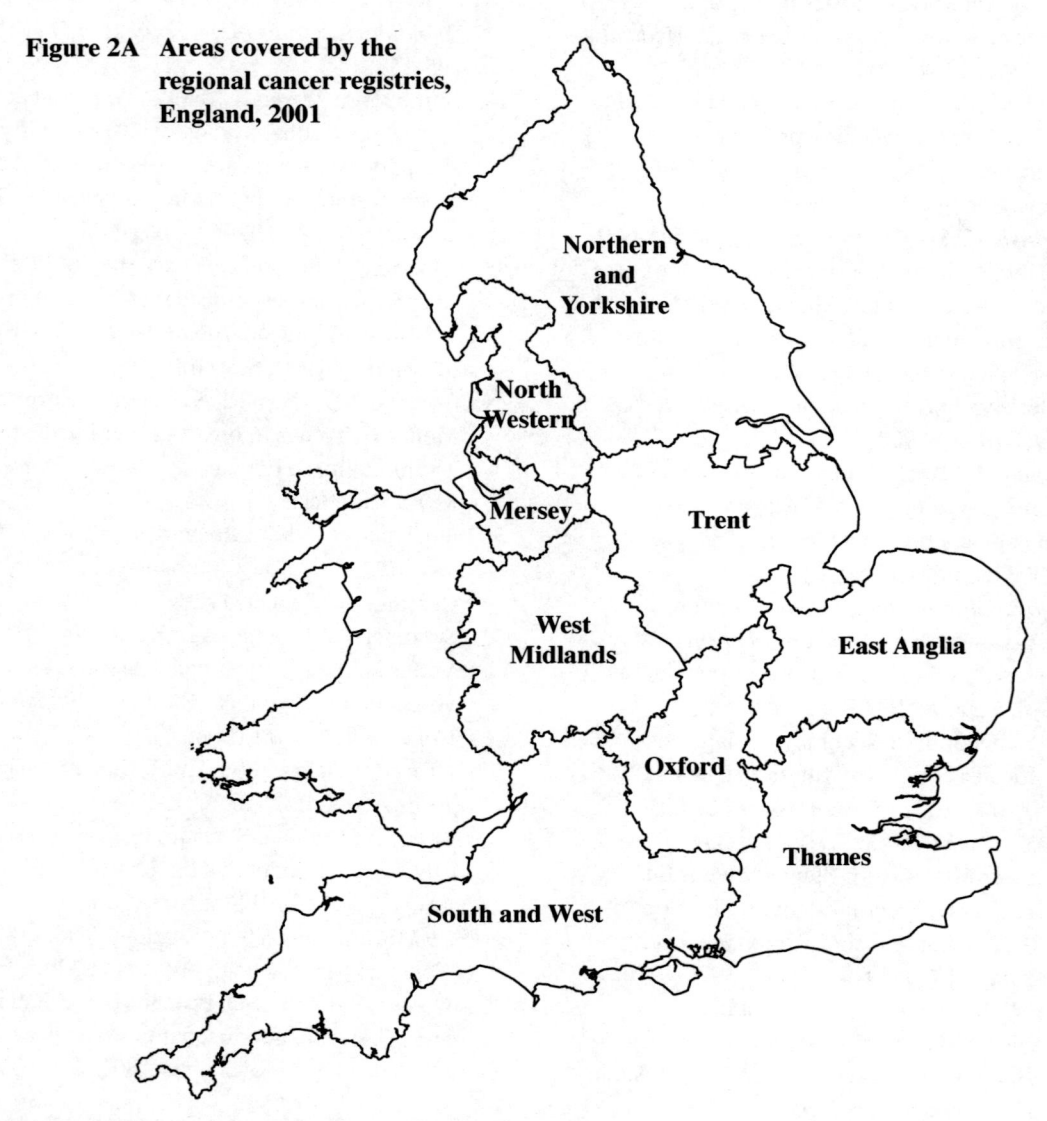

Figure 2A Areas covered by the regional cancer registries, England, 2001

Cancer registries in the United Kingdom:
current directors, addresses, telephone and fax numbers

United Kingdom Association of Cancer Registries website: www.ukacr.org.uk

(a) England

Northern & Yorkshire

Professor R Haward, Medical Director

Tel: 0113 392 4163
Fax: 0113 392 4178
bob.haward@nycris.leedsth.nhs.uk

Professor D Forman,
Director of Information and Research

Tel: 0113 392 4309
Fax: 0113 392 4178
david.forman@nycris.leedsth.nhs.uk

Northern and Yorkshire Cancer Registry and Information Service,
Arthington House
Cookridge Hospital
LEEDS, LS16 6QB

Trent

Post vacant

Trent Cancer Registry
Weston Park Hospital
Whitham Road
SHEFFIELD, S10 2SJ

Tel: 0114 226 3560
Fax: 0114 226 3561

East Anglian

Dr J Rashbass, Director
Dr C Brown, Medical Director

East Anglian Cancer Registry
Box 193,
Level 5 Oncology
Addenbrooke's Hospital
Hills Road
CAMBRIDGE, CB2 2QQ

Tel: 01223 216644
Fax: 01223 245636
eacr@medschl.cam.ac.uk

Figure 2B Areas covered by the government offices for the regions, England, 2001

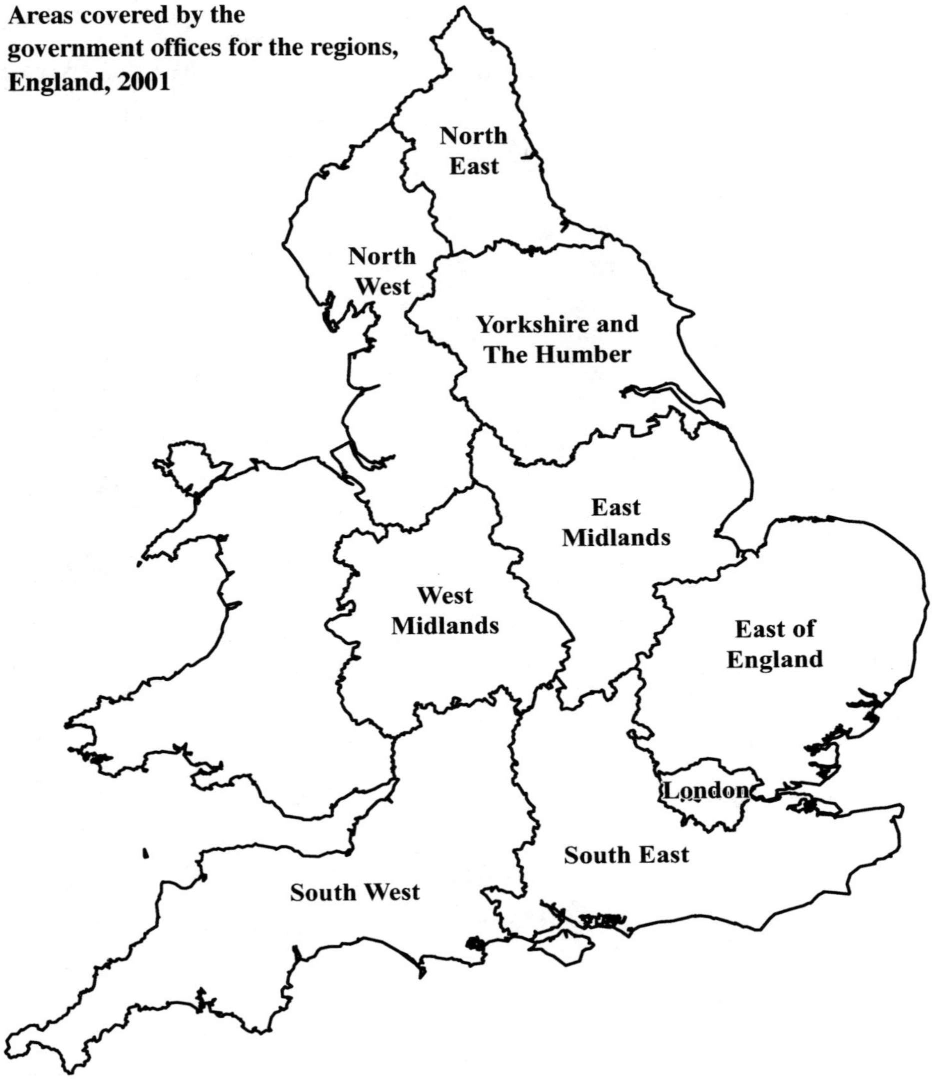

Thames	Cancer Intelligence Unit University of Cambridge Strangeways Research Laboratory Wort's Causeway CAMBRIDGE CB1 8RN Tel: 01223 740273 Email: sara.godward@srl.cam.ac.uk Professor H Møller, Director & Professor of Epidemiology Thames Cancer Registry 1st Floor Capital House 42 Weston Street LONDON, SE1 3QD Tel: 020 7378 7688 Fax: 020 7378 9510 henrik.moller@kcl.ac.uk	Oxford South & West	Dr M Roche, Medical Director Oxford Cancer Intelligence Unit 4150 Chancellor Court Oxford Business Park South OXFORD OX4 2JY Tel: 01865 334770 Fax: 01865 334794 monica.roche@ociu.nhs.uk Dr J Verne, Director South and West Cancer Intelligence Service Grosvenor House 149 Whiteladies Road BRISTOL, BS8 2RA Tel: 0117 970 6474 Fax: 0117 970 6481 jverne.gosw@go-regions.gsi.gov.uk

	Mr T Malik, Deputy Director	**(b) Wales**
	South and West Cancer Intelligence Service Highcroft Romsey Road WINCHESTER, SO22 5DH	Dr J Steward, Director Welsh Cancer Intelligence & Surveillance Unit 14 Cathedral Road CARDIFF, CF11 9LJ
	Tel: 01962 863511 Ext: 3584 Fax: 01962 878360 tmalik@swcis.nhs.uk	Tel: 029 20 373500 Fax: 029 20 373511 john.steward@velindre-tr.wales.nhs.uk
West Midlands	Dr G Lawrence, Director	**(c) Scotland**
	West Midlands Cancer Intelligence Unit Public Health Building The University of Birmingham Edgbaston BIRMINGHAM, B15 2TT	Dr D Brewster, Director of Cancer Registration in Scotland Scottish Cancer Registry Epidemiology and Statistics Group Information Services 1st Floor, Gyle Square 1 South Gyle Crescent EDINBURGH EH12 9EB
	Tel: 0121 415 8129 Fax: 0121 414 7712 gill.lawrence@wmciu.nhs.com	
Merseyside & Cheshire	Dr E M I Williams, Director	
	Merseyside & Cheshire Cancer Registry 2nd Floor Muspratt Building The University of Liverpool LIVERPOOL, L69 3GB	Tel: 0131 275 6092 Fax: 0131 275 7511 david.brewster@isd.csa.scot.nhs.uk **(d) N Ireland**
	Tel: 0151 794 5690 0151 794 5691 Registry Fax: 0151 794 5700 lyn.williams@mccr.nhs.uk	Dr A Gavin, Director Northern Ireland Cancer Registry Dept of Epidemiology & Public Health The Queen's University of Belfast Mulhouse Building Grosvenor Road BELFAST, BT12 6BJ
North Western	Dr A Moran, Director	
	North Western Cancer Registry Centre for Cancer Epidemiology Christie Hospital NHS Trust Kinnaird Road Withington MANCHESTER, M20 9QL	Tel: 028 9063 2573 Fax: 028 9024 8017 a.gavin@qub.ac.uk
	Tel: 0161 446 3566 Fax: 0161 446 3590 tony.moran@cce.man.ac.uk	